S·T·R·E·T·C·H & R·E·L·A·X

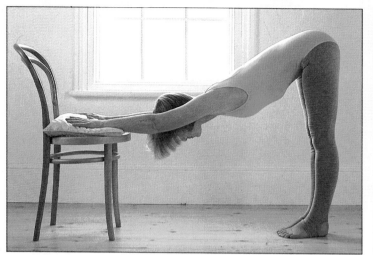

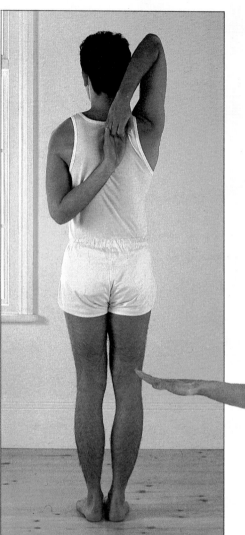

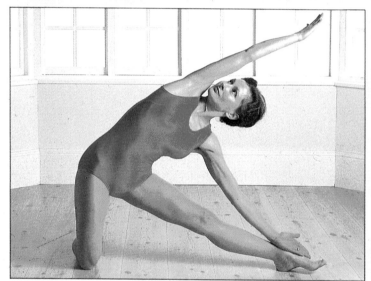

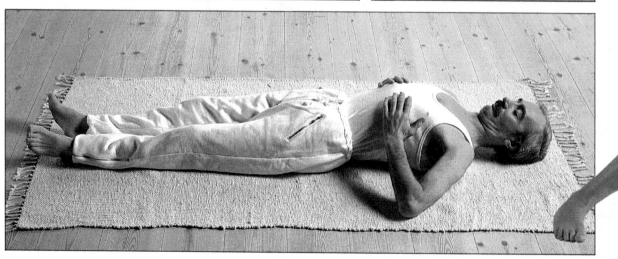

S·T·R·E·T·C·H
&
R·E·L·A·X

·MAXINE TOBIAS· & ·MARY STEWART·

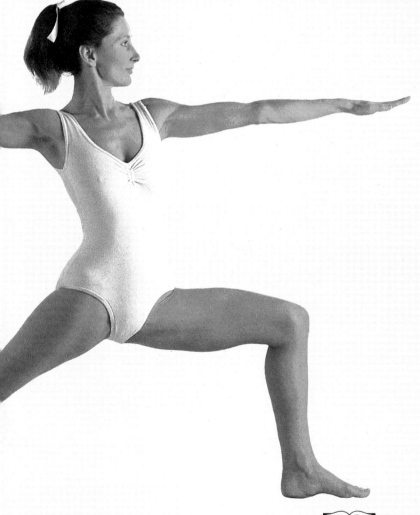

DORLING KINDERSLEY
LONDON • NEW YORK • SYDNEY • MOSCOW

First published in Great Britain in 1985 by
Dorling Kindersley Publishers Limited,
9 Henrietta Street, London WC2E 8PS

Editor: Sybil del Strother
Art editor: Jane Owen

Senior art editor: Anne-Marie Bulat
Managing editor: Daphne Razazan

Photography: Jeff Veitch

British Library Cataloguing in Publication Data

Tobias, Maxine

Stretch and relax
1. Relaxation
I. Title   II. Stewart, Mary
613.7′9   RA790.5

ISBN 0-86318-112-0
ISBN 0-86318-115-5   Pbk

Typeset by Chambers Wallace, London.
Printed in Italy by Arnoldo Mondadori, Verona.

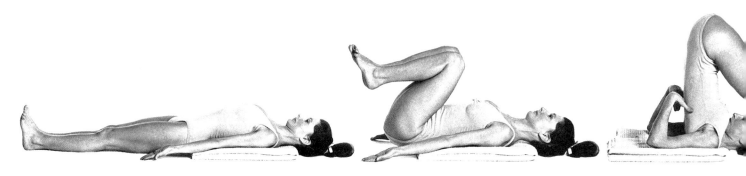

· CONTENTS ·

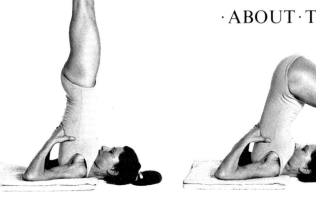
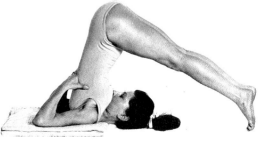
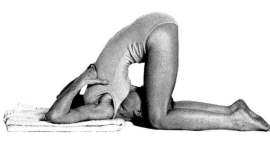

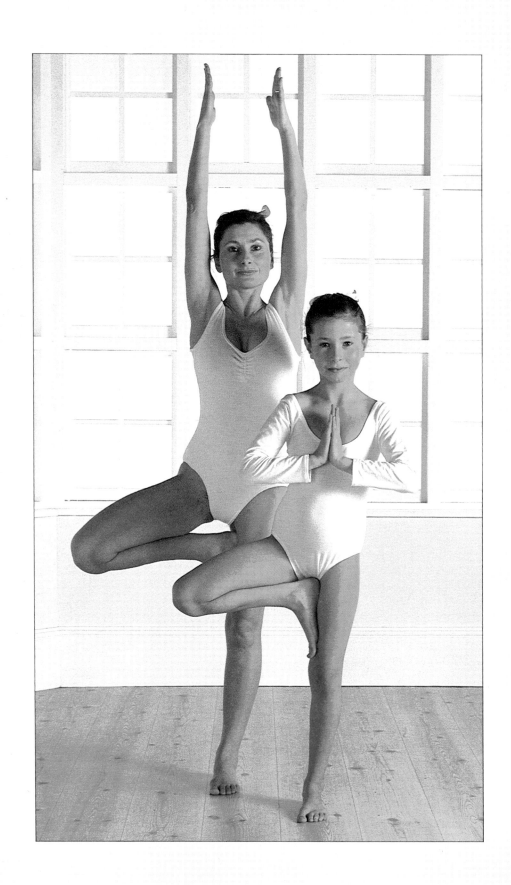

·FOREWORD·

As Health Editor of Vogue between 1979 and 1984, it fell to me to do the rounds of new exercise classes. It was boomtime then and every week at least one new club would contact me, seeking coverage and a few coveted lines in the magazine. As I could only check them by taking part in the classes, I worked out while I worked. Being unfit anyway, I welcomed any chance of getting into shape and flung myself happily into my research. Unfortunately, my enthusiasm soon wore off. The stultifying boredom of repetitious exercise, the aching muscles and debilitating stiffness that would always strike afterwards, and the body that just didn't seem to be getting any stronger or fitter for all the sweating and stretching and grinding I did, left me feeling tired, sore and discouraged. Inside I felt dissatisfied, because outside I was still not the shape I wanted. Surely, there had to be a better way?

There was – but, being the oldest system of exercise around and not the newest, it had escaped my notice. I had heard of yoga, of course, and knew people had been practising it for centuries, but I thought of it as an eastern package demanding a guru, endless time, beautiful thoughts and a working knowledge of Sanskrit. None of which I had or wanted to acquire. And then I had seen those pictures of people turning themselves into pretzels . . . No, it was not for me. Such was my resistance that, although I first met Maxine Tobias in the spring of 1980, it took me three years to take up her invitation and go to a class.

When I did, it was a revelation. Here were all sorts of people of varied ages and abilities working together, each aware of their different capabilities and limitations and each working within them. There was no pressure to do anything people felt was beyond them, no whiff of competition. Instead of barking instructions from the front, as so many other teachers did, Maxine wandered among us making suggestions and adjusting postures, sharing the benefits of her knowledge and expertise. It took just one class for me to realize that I had found the perfect system for me: an approach that was practical and sane, a philosophy that I could take (or leave) at any level and a way of working that actually increased confidence in

my body rather than smashing it to pieces. Far from it being the stiff ungainly object that was forever letting me down, I found that my body was strong, dynamic, capable of far more than I had ever imagined. It was just a matter of working *with* it rather than pitting myself *against* it. The body that had so resolutely refused to do one more press-up or run another lap responded as if by magic – unfolding, stretching, releasing further and further and *further*. I left those early classes feeling exhilarated beyond anything, and at the same time relaxed. My assistant, Joanna, caught my enthusiasm and started classes with Mary. Before long she, too, was drifting into work in a delicious state of calm, feeling more rested and revitalized than she'd been for a long time.

As the months go by, I have new insights. Using the self-awareness that yoga teaches, I now judge my progress by sensing what is happening inside me – my ligaments, joints and muscles (that sensation of what stretch actually *feels* like) – rather than relying on a mirror as my guide. Although my body has become firmer and more toned as a result of practising yoga, the real change has been in the perception of my shape. I feel much friendlier towards my body, I actually like the way it is. I don't think of yoga as "exercise" any more either but as a useful resource that I employ to achieve the results I want – to become stronger and fitter, calmer and less frantic. I carry on with it because it works and the benefits are carried into many different areas of the everyday.

I cannot think of a better way to start bringing some of the benefits of yoga into your life than by following Maxine and Mary's guidance. Use this book, share their knowledge, absorb some of their deep understanding of the way the body works and you will find yoga as exciting an introduction to the amazing things you are capable of as I found in those first classes over two years ago.

Deborah Hutton, 1985

· INTRODUCTION ·

Stretch and Relax is based on yoga, which we both practise and teach. Yoga has never been primarily a method of keeping fit, although health and mental stability are the results of yoga practised correctly. Because *Stretch and Relax* is based on this ancient system, it is not intended to make you conform to a particular standard of physical fitness or a fashionable look. Instead you should find yourself at ease with your body as you strengthen your muscles and improve your posture. Practised regularly, the *Stretch and Relax* system promotes good health, whatever your physical type: it increases your stamina, it reduces fatigue and, above all, it makes you more resistant to stress and minor physical ailments.

· ENJOY · STRETCHING · EVERY · DAY ·

You may occasionally be inspired to start a fitness programme by some fantasy image of how you would like to look or behave. The probability is that all too soon reality catches up with you, and you give up, disheartened and disillusioned. Alternatively, perhaps you hurt your body by forcing it to conform to an unrealistic ideal. This book is based, not on an unreal fantasy, but on the practical needs of men and women in their everyday lives. The stretches, relaxation and breathing can be started by anyone at any time in life. *Stretch and Relax* is not a rigid discipline designed to punish your body, but an enjoyable way of releasing tensions and improving your health through an evolving method that you can tailor to suit your individual needs.

The people who come to the regular classes that we teach are from all walks of life and do all kinds of jobs. The main thing they have in common is that they lead busy lives, without much time for themselves. Working with them over the years, we have seen that those who practise regularly, if only for a few minutes a day, derive much more benefit than those who only attend a class for a weekly workout. Regular practice is therefore the basis of *Stretch and Relax*.

· ANYONE · CAN · STRETCH ·

But practising regularly is not always easy. You need to be motivated by a positive attitude towards your body and its use. Over the years many students have asked us for a daily programme that would help them start practising when they least felt like doing so. As a result we have devised a system of graded stretches, designed to be an enjoyable way of taking your body through the full range of physical movements. The system can be followed by anyone, from stiff beginners to gymnasts. As long as you practise regularly and sensibly, you can adapt the system as your flexibility improves. This means that your practice progresses and does not become dull or stale.

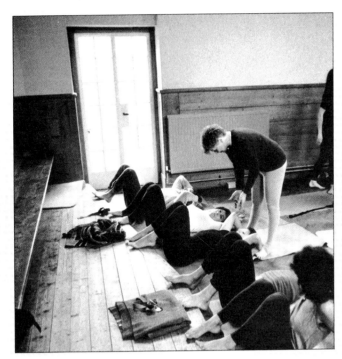

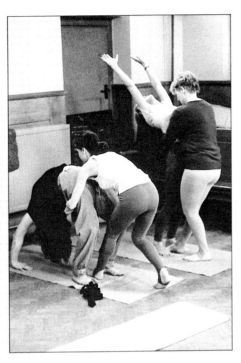

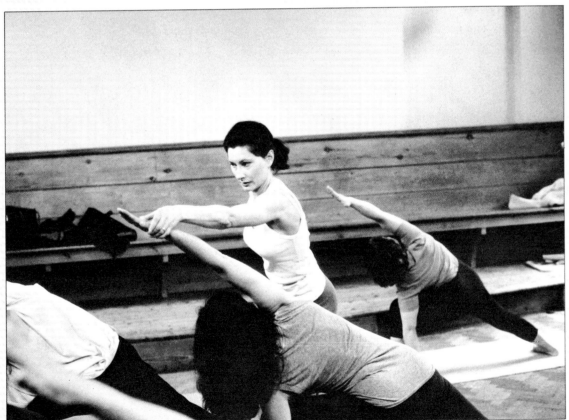

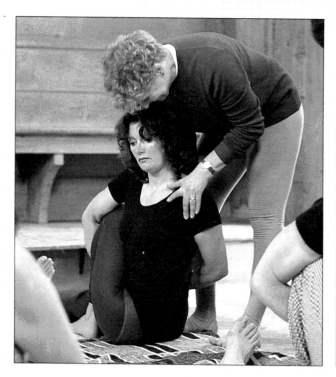

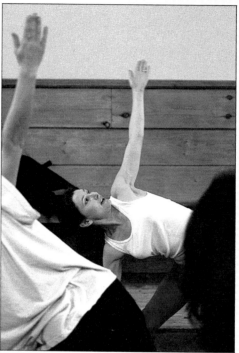

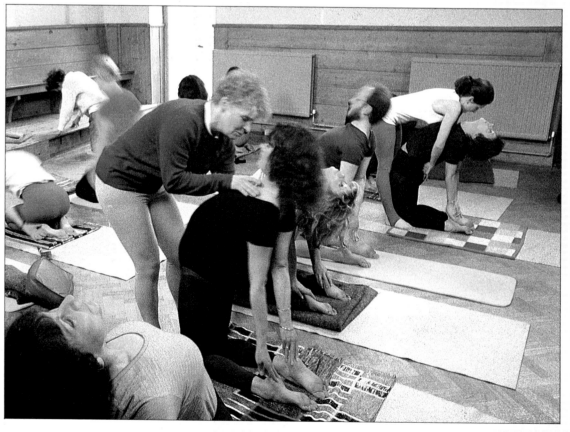

Although the stretches are graded, this does not turn the book into a ladder of excellence which you have to climb. *Stretch and Relax* should be a pleasure to do, bringing a feeling of revitalized energy each time you practise. If you are elderly or stiff you will benefit as much from the "less stretch" movements as the younger and more supple will from extending a bit further. Anyone, from grandparent to grandchild, can practise *Stretch and Relax* and enjoy it.

·STRETCH·IS·NATURAL·

As you adapt to the demands of modern life, you acquire tensions and stiffnesses. Even sportsmen and keep-fit enthusiasts seldom use the full range of their bodies' possible movements. Over the years natural posture is pulled out of alignment by habitual muscular tensions, and your capacity for standing upright and balanced to allow free movement with minimum effort is lost. *Stretch and Relax* will help you re-align your posture and aid your natural ability to adapt to your surroundings, as well as keeping fatigue at bay. It works in harmony with your natural gifts of re-adjustment and recuperation, rather than imposing something alien or difficult on your body.

·RELAX·AFTER·STRETCHING·

Stretching and relaxation go together: when you stretch your body, you feel ready to relax afterwards; as you concentrate on the movements and understand what you are doing, you also calm down. Relaxation is an essential part of daily life. When you practise the stretches you begin to understand the meaning of relaxation, as muscular tension releases. When you finish stretching the natural conclusion is to lie down quietly and give yourself a few minutes of stillness.

·BE·AWARE·OF·YOUR·BODY·

Stretch and Relax will help you improve your health sensibly by becoming aware of your own body and how it is constructed. It will show you how to improve your body's performance and will encourage you to help yourself with minor physical and emotional problems. It is not about getting thin through exercise and we do not include any diets or arduous regimes. However, we do want men and women to think about their bodies constructively, so that they feel good and look good.

We all need high levels of energy to cope with the multiple pressures of modern life. We can all benefit from learning how to use our bodies with the maximum efficiency for the least expenditure of energy. *Stretch and Relax* will help you achieve this.

· HOW · TO · USE · THIS · BOOK ·

This book tells you how to stretch and relax. Used properly it
will serve you for many years. It is a book to work and live
with, not just to read from beginning to end.
The first three chapters are the key to the system.
The rest of the book uses the basic stretch system
for several different purposes.

· STRETCH ·
(pages 14-47)

In this chapter the stretches are explained in
detail. Each basic stretch has alternatives: "less
stretch" movements for those who are stiff or who
are beginners; "more stretch" positions for those
who have practised for some time and who are
supple. Make sure that you are following the
precise instructions for each stretch, especially
when you first start to practise.

· RELAX ·
(pages 48-57)

Relaxation is discussed here. If you find the classic
position for relaxation described on pages 50-1
uncomfortable or unsuitable, there are alternative
positions on pages 52-3. Once you are used to
relaxing, you may like to include some deep
breathing, as described on pages 54-5.

· STRETCH · PROGRAMMES ·
(pages 58-73)

This chapter combines Chapter One with Chapter
Two to give *Stretch and Relax* programmes for
daily practice. Once you are completely familiar
with the stretches you can use this chapter on its
own as a quick guide. There are five different
twenty-minute programmes, for daily use
according to your age and physical ability. There
are also two longer programmes for occasional use.

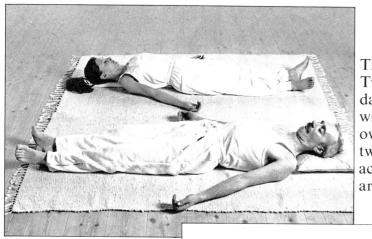

·STRETCH·TOGETHER·
(pages 74-89)

This is a lighthearted look at how to enjoy stretch with your family or friends. You may take it in turns, or you can simply stretch together.

·RELIEVING·STIFFNESS·
(pages 90-113)

You may find certain stretches difficult because some part of your body is particularly stiff. Special stretches to loosen stiffness are given in this chapter. Ideally you should do them daily for as long as your problem persists, immediately before your regular practice programme.

·RELIEVING·STRESS·
(pages 114-27)

This chapter is a little bit different, as it is not about regular routine. As you practise *Stretch and Relax,* you will discover that extending your body can have a profound effect on the way you feel mentally. This chapter suggests ways of applying the technique to help you surmount crises in your life brought on by stress.

·HAVING·A·BABY·
(pages 128-43)

Chapter Seven can help you before, during and after the birth. The stretches develop naturally from the routines set out earlier in the book.

·STRETCH·FURTHER·
(pages 144-55)

The last chapter is to give you a taste of what you can do after you have mastered all the other stretches and programmes in the book. Practice should develop over the years so that it never becomes stale. Here you have a chance to see what can be achieved, preferably with the help of a teacher, by those who have practised *Stretch and Relax* for some years and who fully understand the movements in the simpler stretches.

Remember that it is more important to develop a regular pattern of practice and to understand its effects than it is to attempt the more difficult stretches, so there is no hurry – or even need – to reach the end of the book.

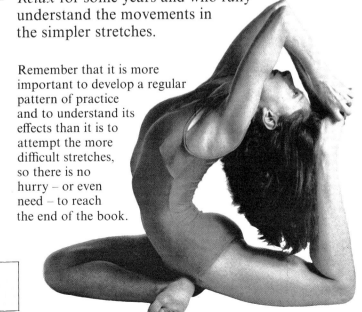

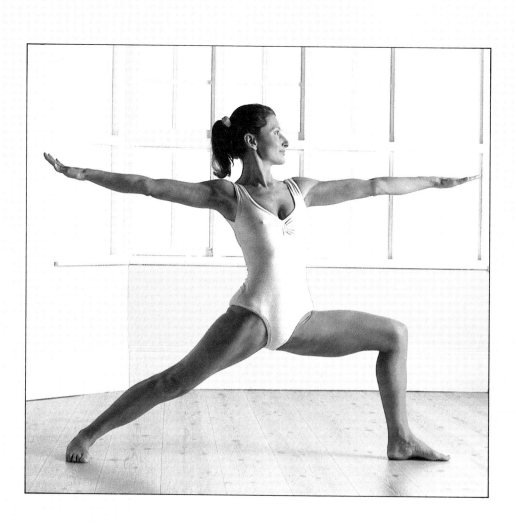

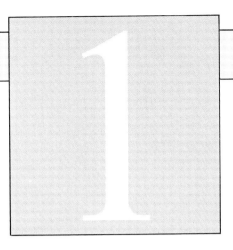

·STRETCH·

The desire to stretch is a natural impulse – you stretch to relieve tiredness or stiffness after being in one position too long. As a form of exercise stretching is easy, enjoyable and safe, the perfect antidote to physical and mental tension. Stretch is good for your entire body, above all for the spine. It releases tightness in the muscles. It improves circulation and relieves stress, leaving you fresh and relaxed. By practising regularly you will not only undo recent muscle tensions but, gradually, long-standing ones as well, so that slowly your posture and your whole range of movement will improve.

Stretch is, however, far more than the undoing of tension. It is the dynamic extension of the muscles, while you focus your attention on the movement of your entire body, rather than just working on a particular group of muscles or a particular joint. This concentration brings insight and awareness of the way your body moves, and you will find your physical, mental and emotional energy reviving.

Breathing deeply is part of stretching. When you stretch to relieve fatigue, you tend to yawn at the same time, taking a deep breath in followed by an out-breath at the end of the stretch. This link between the movement of your body and your breath is developed when you stretch regularly. Take care not to hold your breath and to breathe slowly and evenly. After a while breathing as you stretch will come naturally.

Each of the seven stretches in this chapter is designed to stretch and strengthen your spine, thereby energizing your entire body. The order in which you practise the stretches is important. Not only do the opposing movements have to counter each other, but the strong outward stretches must be balanced by more centred positions. You should therefore learn the stretches in the order in which they appear in this chapter and practise each stretch every day. Once you are familiar with them, you can put them together into programmes (see Chapter Three).

The intensity of the stretch will vary enormously from one individual to the next, and it is important to understand that keeping your body supple and relaxed is not a competition. In fact, however fit and flexible you are, you should start with the "less stretch" movements to ensure you are feeling and understanding the stretches correctly. Regularity of practice, not intensity of practice, is the key to success.

·GENERAL·POINTS·

Read the following points before you start to stretch.
They are important if you want to stretch in complete safety
and get the most out of your practice.

1 If you are healthy, you can stretch. The simple "less stretch" variations of the basic positions should be possible for anyone to do. If you have any doubts at all, take medical advice before you start to practise.

2 Go slowly. If you decide to follow the basic programme, learn the "less stretch" positions for each stretch first, so that your body gets used to the correct movements. The "more stretch" positions demand strength and flexibility. Even if you have been doing other forms of physical exercise and your body is already very supple when you start stretching, you should practise the basic stretches daily for some months before you try anything more advanced.

3 Practise the stretches in the order in which they are presented. Try to learn them in sequence, not picking out one or two in isolation.

4 In many of these positions you keep your legs straight. To prevent yourself from pushing into the backs of your knees and injuring your ligaments, pull up your kneecaps by tightening your front thigh muscles.

5 Wear loose clothing, whatever feels comfortable. Leotards and tights are not essential.

6 Work on a non-slip surface with bare feet so that you can stretch your toes for maximum contact with the floor.

7 Do not practise immediately after eating.

8 Rest when your body is tired. Your stamina will increase as you practise regularly.

9 Relax your muscles and never force your body into a stretch. As you extend your limbs, your muscles elongate away from your spine, enabling your joints to move freely.

10 Go into each movement on an out-breath and then breathe normally. Do not hold your breath, as this causes tension and strain. As you come up out of the stretch, breathe in.

11 Jump your feet into position, when you need to take them wide apart. If you are pregnant or elderly, however, it is probably more sensible simply to step into position. The instructions suggest how far apart you should take your feet. These distances are only approximate and may be varied according to your height.

12 Hold each stretch for as long as you can comfortably continue releasing your muscles. At first this will be only a few seconds, but as you begin to practise regularly the time you can hold the position will gradually increase.

13 Be conscious of the way your spine moves as you stretch. Feel the movement along the back of your body as well as the front. If this is difficult ask someone to help you with a pole (see Chapter Four).

14 Do each side stretch on both sides, holding the position on the second side for the same length of time as on the first. You may find you tend to stretch more on your stronger side; make sure you work on both sides evenly.

15 Come up out of the positions with as much care as you go into them. To come out of a stretch, repeat the movements you used to go into it, in reverse order. You should take especial care with the upside down positions (see pages 42-7), as coming out of them too fast could put excessive strain on the vertebrae of the neck.

· STRAIGHT ·

Stretching your spine up, against the pull of gravity, allows your whole body to move freely and easily. Take some trouble following the instructions below, and you will feel the benefit as you do the outward stretches.

Start from your feet

Stand with the outer edges of your bare feet parallel to each other and your big toes touching. You may have to keep your heels slightly apart. Stretch your toes fully as they help to balance and support your trunk. (If you have bunions or deformed toes you may find this difficult – see pages 112-13.) From the balls of your feet extend back into your heels. Your weight should be taken evenly on the arches of both feet, and you should feel your feet firm and stable on the floor.

Lift up from your arches and stretch up through your legs, pulling up your kneecaps by tightening your front thigh muscles. The backs of your knees should also extend, but do not push back into them as this could strain your calf muscles. Tighten the muscles underneath your buttocks so that your coccyx (tailbone) feels "tucked in". When held correctly the pelvis is horizontal, not tilted either backwards or forwards (see page 93), and in this position it gives the spine maximum support.

Stretch up through your spine

As you stretch up from your pelvis, the muscles of your abdomen act to help your lumbar spine extend and stop it sagging inwards. This relieves pressure on the lower back. Lift your ribcage at the back as well as the front and feel the muscles of the back of the chest stretch away from your spine. This is known as opening the chest. Make space between your hips and your ribs.

Stretch your arms up above your head, feeling the lift in your spine. Then drop them by your side again, without losing the spinal stretch. Drop your shoulders. Do not tense them to feel more lift. Hold your arms loosely and use their weight to help your shoulders drop.

Extend your neck up into the base of your skull without lifting your chin or pulling it in too far. Feel as if you are being pulled up by the crown of your head. Your whole body should feel firm but light, while you breathe smoothly and easily.

From this basic standing stretch, your body is free to move in all directions.

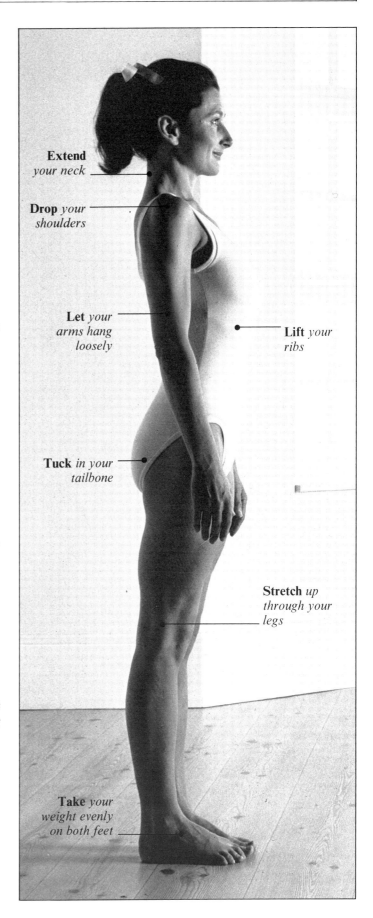

Extend *your neck*

Drop *your shoulders*

Let *your arms hang loosely*

Tuck *in your tailbone*

Lift *your ribs*

Stretch *up through your legs*

Take *your weight evenly on both feet*

·SIDEWAYS·

In these stretches you extend the whole of the spine to the side, so keeping your hips and spine flexible. It is a movement you should practise regularly, especially since as you get older you don't move like this often in your daily activities.

The firm stretch of the legs allows the lower spine to release, relieving low backache. At the same time outstretched arms and the extension of the back of the neck keep the upper spine mobile.

If your hips are stiff when you start to practise, you may try to go down too far, bending from the waist instead of from the hips. Your trunk will then drop forward and you will lose the sideways stretch in the lower back. In order to get used to the correct stretch in the hips and lower back, practise the "less stretch" positions on page 20 first. Page 78 will also help you with the correct alignment of this position.

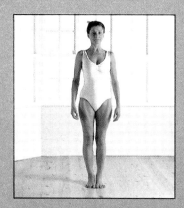 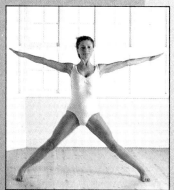 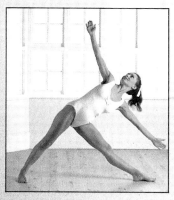

1 Stand tall and stretch up through your spine. With your feet together, spread out your toes and pull up from your arches. Pull up your kneecaps and stretch your whole spine. Extend your neck and relax your face.

2 Take your feet 1m (3ft) apart, keeping them parallel. Maintain the lift of your spine so that your chest is open and your shoulders are relaxed. Stretch out your arms, with the palms of your hands facing the floor.

3 Turn your right foot slightly in and your left leg out to the side, lining up your left heel with the arch of your right foot. Pull up your kneecaps. Breathing out, move your hips to the right and extend your spine sideways to the left.

Pull *up your kneecaps and keep your back leg strong*

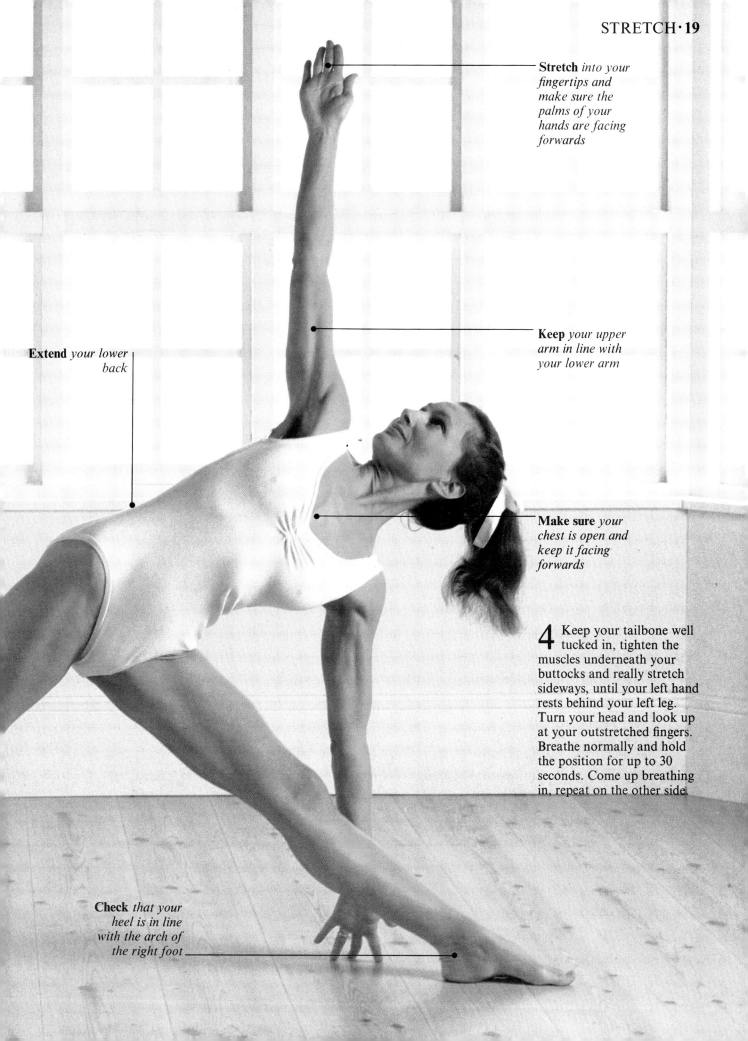

Stretch *into your fingertips and make sure the palms of your hands are facing forwards*

Keep *your upper arm in line with your lower arm*

Extend *your lower back*

Make sure *your chest is open and keep it facing forwards*

4 Keep your tailbone well tucked in, tighten the muscles underneath your buttocks and really stretch sideways, until your left hand rests behind your left leg. Turn your head and look up at your outstretched fingers. Breathe normally and hold the position for up to 30 seconds. Come up breathing in, repeat on the other side.

Check *that your heel is in line with the arch of the right foot*

·SIDEWAYS·
LESS STRETCH

The stiffer you are the more important it is to get a
good stretch before you go sideways. The stretches
on this page will release stiffness, especially in the
hips. If you have the sensation of dropping
forwards, practise with your back against a wall.

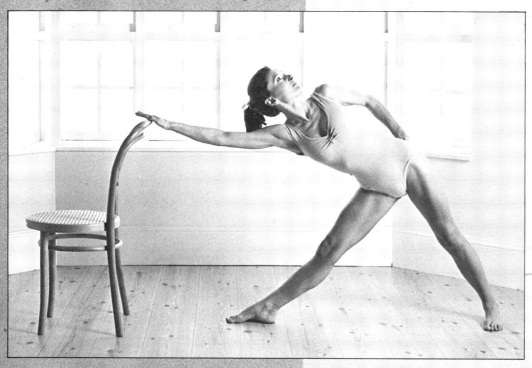

First stretch
Place a chair to your right.
Take your feet about 1m
(3ft) apart and stretch your
arms out. Turn your left foot
slightly in, your right leg out
as on pp. 18-19. Put your
left hand on your hip and
stretch to the right without
dropping forwards. Keep
your chest open and really
stretch your lower spine.
Hold for a few seconds,
breathe in and come up.
Repeat on the other side.

Second stretch
Stand tall and stretch up
through your spine. Take
your feet 1m (3ft) apart and
stretch out your arms. Turn
your left foot slightly in and
your right leg out. Breathe
out and put your right hand
on your leg, stretching to the
right without bending
forwards. Hold for a few
seconds, breathe in, come
up. Repeat on the other side.

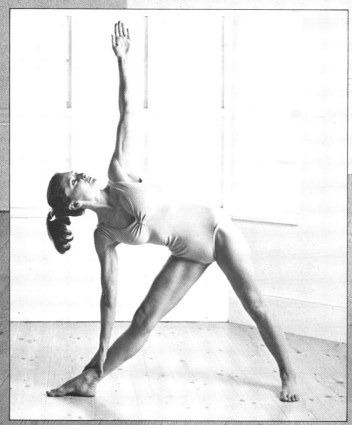

· SIDEWAYS ·
MORE STRETCH

This exhilarating stretch increases flexibility in the hips and spine and tones the muscles in the abdomen and legs. The intense stretch along the upper side of the body loosens the shoulders while the expansion in the chest is good for breathing.

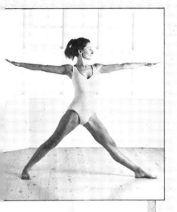

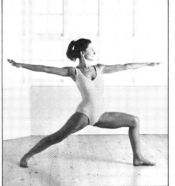

1 Take your feet about 1.5m (4½ft) apart. Turn your right foot in and your left leg out to the side, turning your left thigh out at the hip and pulling up your kneecaps.

2 Keep your right leg firm while you bend your left knee to a right angle. This should be done by lowering your hips so that your left thigh runs parallel to the floor.

3 Breathe out and extend your trunk along your left thigh, taking your left hand down behind your foot and pressing your left knee back against your armpit. Stretch out your right arm over your right ear. Extend your spine to the left. Keep your right shoulder back and look up. Breathe normally as you hold for 20 seconds, then breathe in, come up and repeat on the other side.

·WIDE & STRONG·

These strong and dynamic stretches extend the limbs away from the centre of the body as well as stretching the spine. They loosen the hip joints and tone the leg muscles and so they are very good for athletic people, especially runners. Such invigorating stretches need stability, so your feet should be firm and strong on the floor. Your spine lifts as your arms stretch powerfully, and your breath deepens as your chest expands. At first you will probably be able to hold the stretch comfortably for only a short time, but with continued practice your stamina will increase.

If your hips and shoulders are stiff, practise the "less stretch" positions on page 24 until you feel able to appreciate the fuller stretches.

Extend *your back arm strongly*

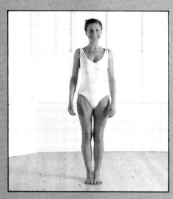 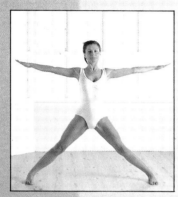 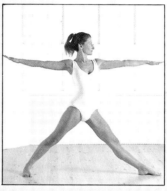

1 Stand tall and straight, with your feet together. Press your feet firmly into the floor. Pull up from your arches and stretch up through your legs and along the curves of your spine. Keep your shoulders down and your facial muscles completely relaxed.

2 Take your feet wide apart (1.3m or 4½ft). Keep the upward stretch in your spine and extend your arms at shoulder level. Stretch away from your trunk into your fingertips, the palms of your hands facing the floor.

3 Turn your right foot slightly in and your left leg out, aligning your left heel with the arch of your right foot. Turn your head to the left and keep the stretch wide and strong. Focus your eyes beyond your fingertips and keep your shoulders relaxed.

4 Breathing out, bend your left knee and take your hips down. Your left thigh should be parallel to the floor with a right angle at the knee. Keep your right leg straight and stretch out strongly from the centre. Hold for up to 30 seconds, come up breathing in, and repeat on the other side.

Keep *the outside of your back foot on the floor*

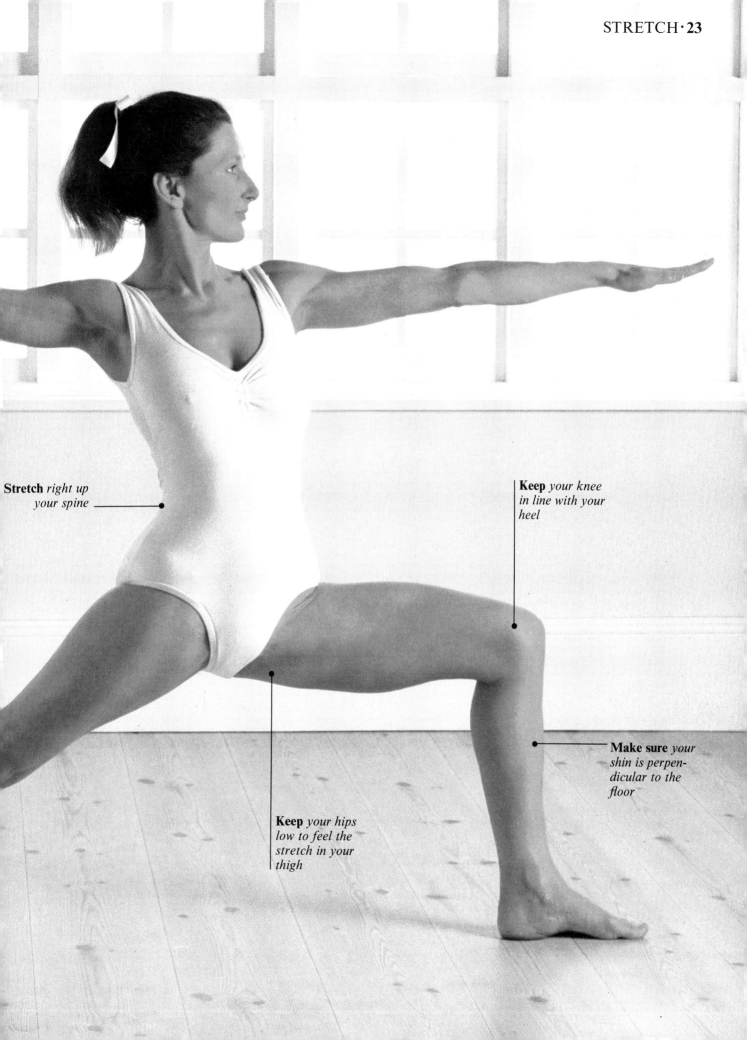

Stretch *right up your spine*

Keep *your knee in line with your heel*

Make sure *your shin is perpendicular to the floor*

Keep *your hips low to feel the stretch in your thigh*

·WIDE & STRONG·
LESS STRETCH

With age the shoulder joints stiffen, making it hard
to extend the body as a whole: the stretches on
this page help keep them flexible, while the upward
stretch of the arms lifts the spine.

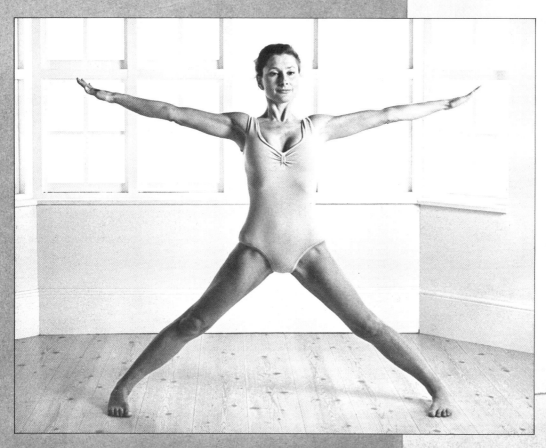

First stretch
Take your feet wide apart,
with your toes pointing
forwards and the arches of
your feet lifted up. Turn
your thighs outwards, knees
straight. Stretch your arms
out strongly from your spine
into your fingertips. You will
feel your breathing deepen as
your chest expands. Hold
for a few seconds.

Second stretch
Stretch your arms out as
above. Breathing out, stretch
your arms straight up above
your head, your palms facing
each other. Keep the
outsides of your feet firmly
on the floor. Take a few deep
breaths, stretching up each
time you breathe out, then
take your arms down.

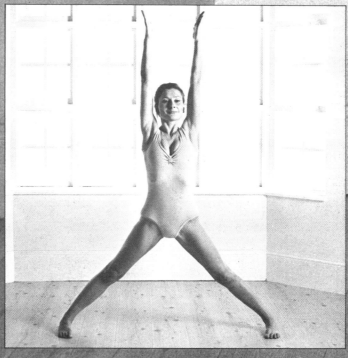

· WIDE & STRONG ·
MORE STRETCH

These advanced stretches require strong back muscles and flexible hips and shoulders. You may find it difficult to balance in the second stretch; if so practise the first position only until you gain confidence. You will then feel able to balance securely on one leg.

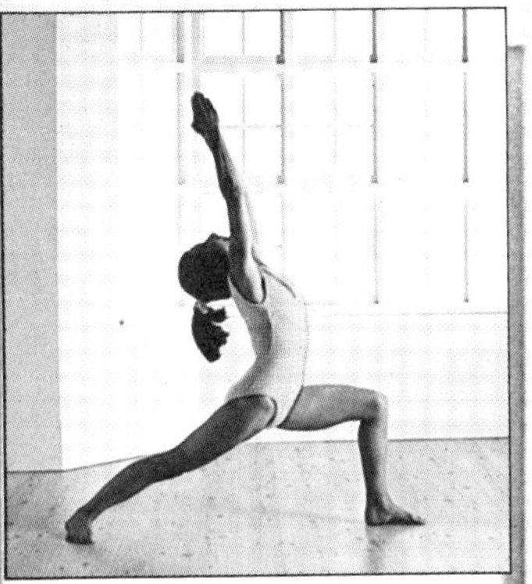

First stretch

Stand with your feet wide apart. Pointing your right foot in and your left leg out, turn completely to the left and stretch your arms up over your head, with your palms facing each other. Lift your back ribs as you stretch into your fingertips. Breathing out, bend your left knee and lower your hips until your left leg makes a right angle at the knee. Breathe normally for up to 20 seconds; then breathe in, come up and repeat on the other side.

Second stretch

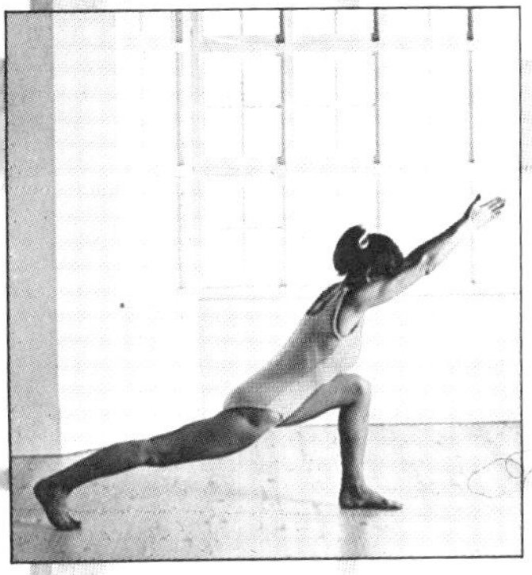

1 Carry on from the last stretch by lifting your back heel, tucking in your tailbone and stretching forwards along your front thigh. Keep your hips well down so that your lower back extends.

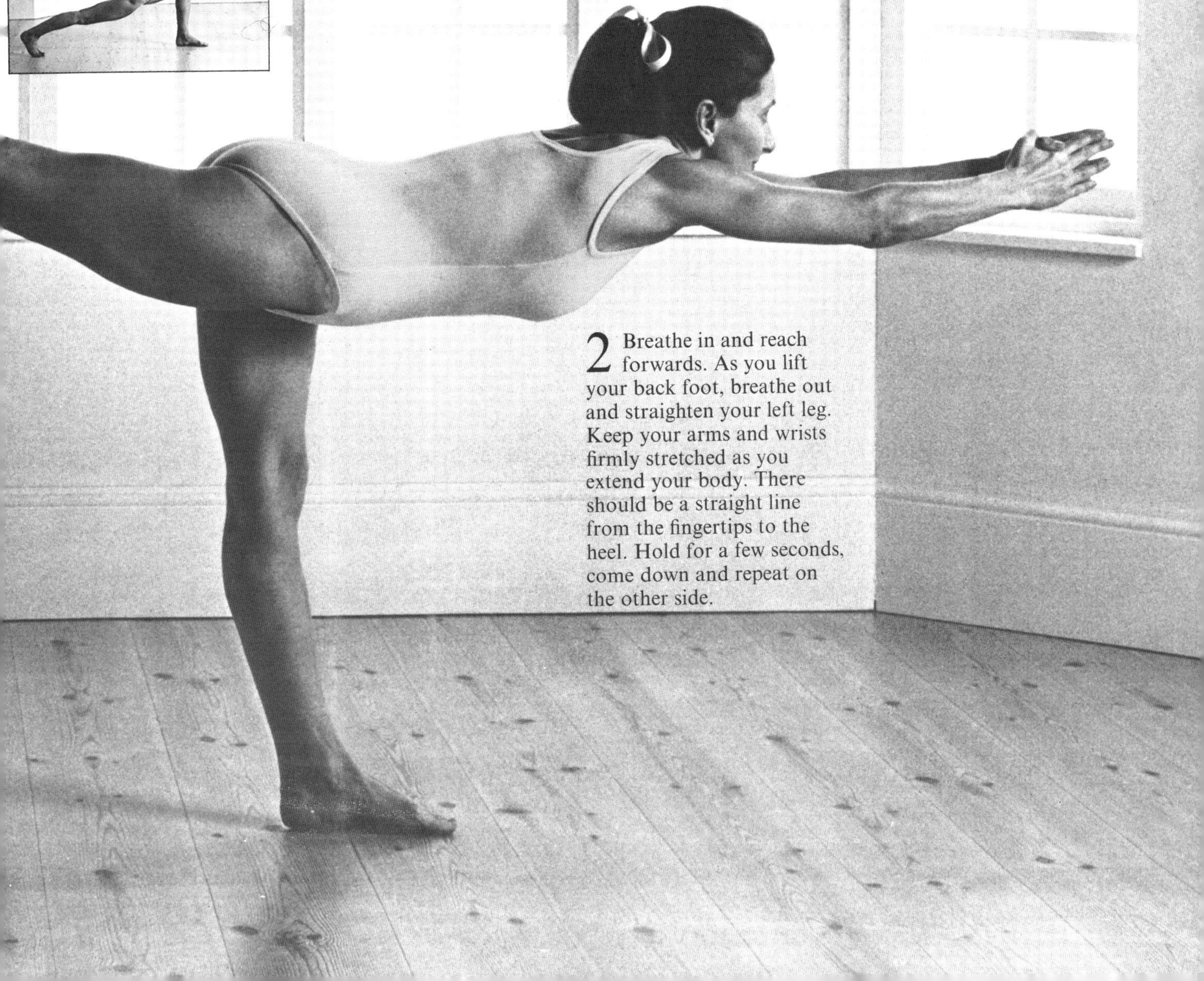

2 Breathe in and reach forwards. As you lift your back foot, breathe out and straighten your left leg. Keep your arms and wrists firmly stretched as you extend your body. There should be a straight line from the fingertips to the heel. Hold for a few seconds, come down and repeat on the other side.

·BACK·TO·THE·CENTRE·

As you do these stretches, your limbs are brought back to the centre of your body after the strong outward movements. This helps you concentrate and induces a feeling of calmness.

Take care to maintain the upward lift of the spine, otherwise you will lose the energizing effect of the outward stretches. Your eyes should stay open, while you look forwards without straining.

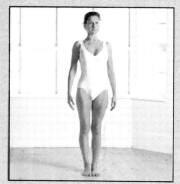 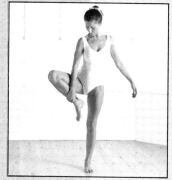 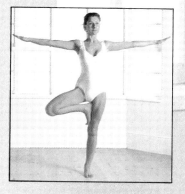

1 Stand up tall and straight with your feet together. Pull up through your legs and stretch along the curves of your spine, keeping your coccyx (tailbone) tucked in and your shoulders relaxed.

2 Bend your right knee and use one or both hands to raise your right leg. Place your right foot as high as possible on the inside of your left thigh, so that your toes are pointing down.

3 Extend your arms at shoulder level and stretch into your fingertips. To help you balance, keep your left leg straight and strong and spread out the toes of your left foot. You should feel firm as you balance on one leg.

4 Keeping your spine straight and your shoulders relaxed, open your chest and bring your palms together. Your right foot should press on your inside left thigh while your left leg stays straight and stable. Take a few deep breaths, repeat on the other side.

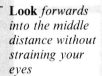

Look *forwards into the middle distance without straining your eyes*

Feel *the even pressure of your palms*

Drop *your shoulders and keep your chest open*

Keep *your hips straight*

Press *your heel as high as possible on your thigh*

Spread *out your toes*

·BACK·TO·THE·CENTRE·
LESS STRETCH

To begin with you may find it difficult to balance steadily on one leg in the basic stretch position. If so, practise the positions on this page for a few months first. They improve flexibility at the hips as well as having a calming effect.

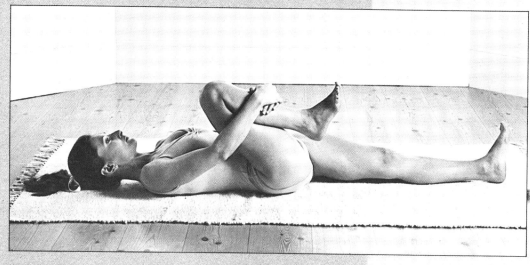

First stretch
Lie down on your back on a rug. Breathing out, bend your right leg and bring it close to your trunk. Keeping your left leg straight, gently pull your right leg towards you until you can hold it round the shin. Your hips should stay flat on the floor. Hold for 30 seconds and repeat on the other side.

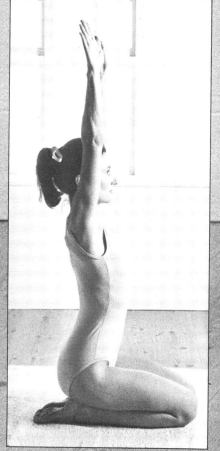

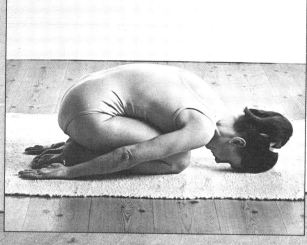

Second stretch

1 Kneel on a thick soft rug or blanket on the floor, sitting on your heels. Link your fingers together, turn your palms outwards and stretch your arms up over your head. Release your fingers. Keep your bottom down on your heels.

2 Bring your arms down close to your thighs and fold your body forwards. Lower your head until it touches the ground. Breathe out as you bend forwards and breathe naturally for about a minute. Then breathe in and come up. Repeat the stretch, again starting with your fingers linked, the opposite thumb on top.

·BACK·TO·THE·CENTRE·
MORE STRETCH

This position is difficult as you need to turn the thighs out at the hips and stretch up at the same time. Most people will have to practise for some months before they feel comfortable doing this.

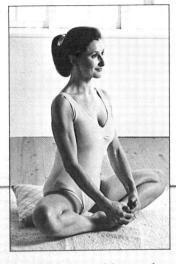

Sit on the floor with your legs straight out in front of you and stretch up, arms behind you and fingers touching the floor. Spread your legs wide, then bend your knees and bring your feet close to your body, soles together. Your thighs should turn out and your knees go down (left). If it is hard to keep your lower back stretching up, raise your hips by sitting on a cushion (above). Hold your feet close in with your hands and stretch along your spine, relaxing your hips further so that your knees go down more. Hold for up to 1 minute.

·FORWARDS·

These stretches are very good for the lower back when they are done correctly. The problem is that the pelvis needs to rotate forwards around the top of the thigh bones if the trunk is to move forwards freely. Many people find the correct rotation hard and compensate by putting extra strain on the spine. If tight back thigh muscles (hamstrings) make the correct rotation difficult, practise the positions on page 32 for several months.

Stand or sit with your weight evenly distributed and make sure that you are straight. Always remember that the movement is *up* and forwards, stretching away from your hips and keeping your chest open so that you can breathe naturally through the stretch. If you have a slipped disc or lumbago (see pages 96-9), do not practise the bending part of these stretches; practise the upward forward movements only.

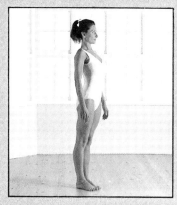 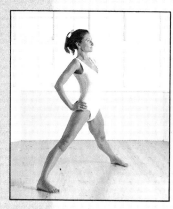 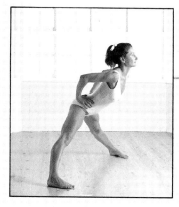

1 Stand tall and straight, with your feet together. Pull up through your legs and stretch along the length of your spine, making your neck long while keeping your shoulders and arms relaxed.

2 Take your feet very wide apart, with your toes pointing forwards and your arches lifted up. Bend your elbows and put your hands squarely on your hips. Lifting from the hips stretch up through your spine.

3 Keeping your legs straight breathe out and stretch forwards from the hips. Do not push into the backs of your knees. Keep your back extended and the weight of your body evenly supported by your feet.

4 Continue to stretch forwards until you can place your hands on the floor in front of you. Pull up the backs of your thighs and extend the front of your trunk forwards and upwards.

Keep *the weight on your feet and press them firmly into the ground*

Extend *your neck without tensing the muscles*

Make sure *your hips stay back in line with your feet*

Take care *not to let your back cave in*

Pull up *through your kneecaps and keep your legs strong and straight*

Keep *your hands shoulder width apart*

·FORWARDS· LESS STRETCH

When you bend forwards you have to bend from the hips as well as stretching the spine. These "less stretch" positions are for people who have tight hamstrings, which prevent the pelvis rotating forwards over the tops of the thigh bones.

First stretch
Put a chair against the wall so it cannot slip. Stand facing it, so that when you go forwards you will touch the chair back. Your feet should be about 30cm (1ft) apart and parallel. Keeping your legs straight, stretch up and forwards from your hips and put your hands on the back of the chair. Breathing out, extend the stretch as far as you can, lengthening the front of your body and keeping your back straight. Your hips should stay in line with your feet. You will feel the stretch in the backs of your thighs. Hold the position for up to 30 seconds. Then breathe in and come up.

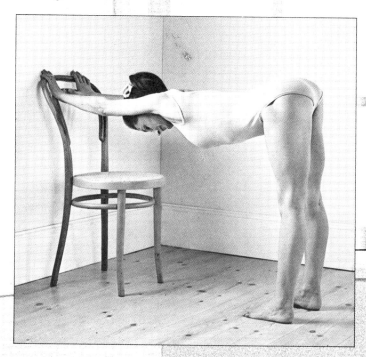

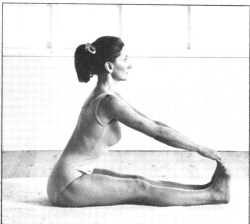

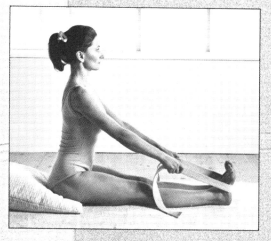

Second stretch
Sit on the floor with your legs straight out in front of you. The weight should be a little to the front of your buttock bones so that you can lift from your lower back. If this is difficult sit on a cushion or folded blanket. Stretch up and forwards so that you can catch your feet (above left). If you collapse at your waist when you do this, loop a belt or tie round your feet and hold that instead (above right). Your legs should stay straight. If they bend, use the belt. Move from the base of your spine and do not pull hard with your hands. Elongate the back of your neck and keep your shoulders relaxed. Hold for as long as you can without strain or tightness (up to 30 seconds), breathing normally. Do not practise the basic stretch until you can do without the belt.

·FORWARDS·
MORE STRETCH

When the pelvis rotates forwards properly you can bend without putting undue strain on the lumbar spine. In these positions you should be able to stretch forwards without straining or pulling with your hands.

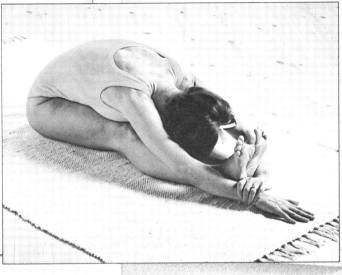

First stretch

Sit on the floor and catch your feet as in the "less stretch" position opposite. Breathing out, stretch the front of your trunk forwards along your thighs. Do not pull with your hands but extend gently from the base of your spine. Then lower your head. Eventually you will be able to hold your hands beyond the soles of your feet and let your shoulders relax. Stay in this position for up to 30 seconds, breathing normally, and then sit up, breathing in. This is a good alternative to the standing stretch (left).

Second stretch

You should attempt this stretch only if the backs of your thighs will extend without strain and you can put your hands on the floor without bending your knees. Stand with your feet together and your legs straight. Raise your arms above your head and stretch up tall. Bring your arms down and bend forwards, breathing out. Extending your spine and keeping your lower back concave for as long as possible, relax your neck. Continue to bend forwards from your hips. The top of your head should move towards your feet; if you are supple you will be able to hold your hands behind your ankles. Stay in the position breathing normally and then come up. Breathing in, extend forwards. Breathe out and stand straight.

·TWIST·

The twisting positions keep the spine flexible as well as helping to release tension in the hips and shoulders. When the movements are done correctly the shoulders move back and down and the top of the spine moves in, so this is an excellent stretch for correcting a rounded back (see page 99).

The thoracic vertebrae of the upper back rotate more freely than the large lumbar vertebrae of the waist. It is therefore important to stretch properly from the lower back and turn the spine completely as you twist rather than just pushing the chest out and turning the ribcage. Because of the upward inward movement of the lower back, twists are very good for lower back pain.

The correct movements can be hard to understand, so start with the "less stretch" positions however supple you are. Throughout your aim is to rotate your body around your straight spine as you stretch up.

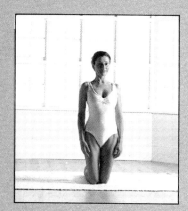 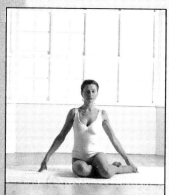 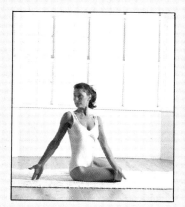

1 Kneel with your knees and feet together. Stretch up along the curves of your spine, keeping your shoulders down. Extend your neck and let your arms relax.

2 Slide your hips to the right and sit on the floor with your legs folded behind you to the left. Keep your left buttock on the ground. If this is difficult you can sit on a small cushion. Lift from your lower back and stretch upwards to the crown of your head.

3 Place your left hand on the outside of your right knee and take your right arm behind you. Breathing out, twist round as far as you can to the right without raising your left hip. Keep your right knee in line with your hip. Keep the fingertips of your right hand on the floor.

4 When you can get a good twist round, hold the back of your left arm with your right hand. Breathing normally, hold the position for 30 seconds, relax and then repeat on the other side.

Make sure *your head stays in line with your hips*

Keep *your neck long*

Open *your chest and keep your shoulders relaxed*

Feel *the stretch in your lower back and make it long*

Keep *both hips down*

Lift *your lower abdomen*

·TWIST·
LESS STRETCH

The stretches on this page are beneficial if you
have stiff joints or a tendency to stoop. They are
particularly useful if you cannot sit in the basic
position on pages 34-5 or if you find it difficult to
lift your lower back.

First stretch
Sit on a chair, your weight
slightly forwards. Do not
collapse the back of your
waist but sit up tall, so that
the front of your body is
stretched and your chest is
open. Then, without moving
your hips, twist to the right
and hold the back of the
chair seat with your right
hand, putting the back of
your left hand against your
right thigh. Keep your knees
in line with your hips. As
you turn, drop your
shoulders, letting your spine
stretch up from the hips.
Hold for 30 seconds, relax
and repeat on the other side.

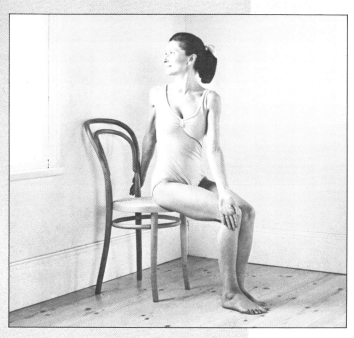

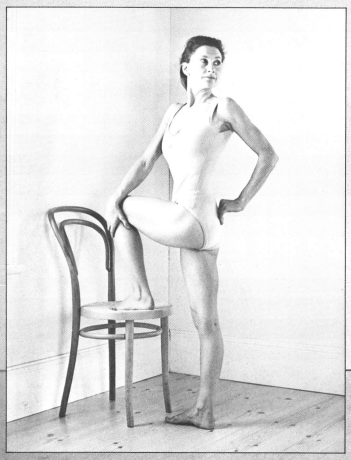

Second stretch
Stand facing a chair, with
your feet pointing straight
ahead. Put your left foot on
the seat, keeping your left
hip down. If you are very
tall, you may have to put a
book on the seat of the chair.
Stand up tall and extend the
front of your body, keeping
your shoulders down and
your chest open. Put your
left hand on the base of your
spine and your right hand
against your left thigh. Then,
without moving your hips,
twist as far round to the left
as you can, looking back
over your left shoulder. Hold
for 30 seconds, relax and
repeat on the other side.

·TWIST·
MORE STRETCH

In these twists you must feel the movement in your lower back. You have to stretch the spine up as you start to turn, keeping it elongated. Because this is difficult when you are sitting with your legs straight out in front of you, do not attempt the second stretch on this page unless you can easily do the "more stretch forwards" positions on page 33.

First stretch
Stand with your feet 1m (3ft) apart and your arms extended. Turn your feet to the left as for the "basic stretch sideways" position (see pp. 18-19). Breathe out and turn from your hips, extending your right arm over your left foot. Open your chest as you stretch your left arm up and out from your trunk. Turn your head to look up at your left hand. Breathing normally, hold the position for as long as you comfortably can; come up and repeat on the other side.

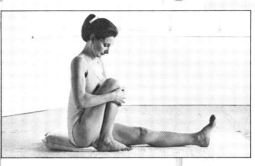

Second stretch
1 Sit with legs straight. Bend your right leg, your heel close to your buttock.

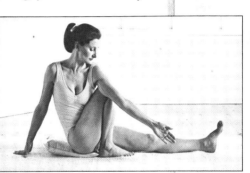

2 With your right hand on the floor behind you, lift up your ribcage so that your lower back goes in and turn as far as possible to the right. Without tensing your abdominal muscles, extend the back of your left arm around the outside of your right knee.

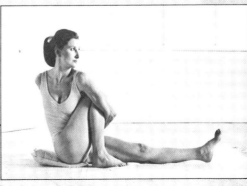

3 Catch your hands behind your back as you turn further. Keep the outside of your right hip down. Hold for up to 20 seconds, relax and repeat on the other side.

·BACKWARDS·

The backward stretch of the spine is a powerful and invigorating movement. Because the extension of the spine works directly on its natural curves, it is important not merely to exaggerate the curve at the waist and neck. Instead you should aim to stretch the spine as a single unit, lengthening the curves and opening the chest and hips. This pose corrects rounded shoulders and prevents the convex curve of the upper spine from becoming too exaggerated (see page 99). Done properly this stretch is the key to youthful posture and vitality.

To extend the spine evenly, strong muscles are needed as well as flexible joints. It is therefore essential that if you are very flexible you should gain strength by practising the "less stretch" positions for a time before you attempt the more difficult backward stretches. If you are uncomfortable with your head back in the basic position because of stiffness in the upper back and neck, the advice again is to practise the "less stretch" positions first.

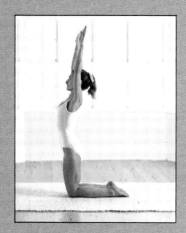 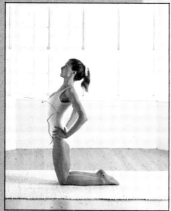 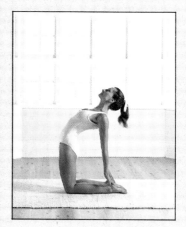

1 Kneel with your feet and knees together and your weight distributed evenly. Stretch your arms above your head in order to lift your spine and back ribs.

2 Move your hands to your hips and continue to stretch up. Keep the back of your waist long. As you begin to curve your spine backwards it is essential to lift and open your chest.

3 Tighten the muscles underneath your buttocks and push your hips forwards so that your thighs stay perpendicular. Stretch your spine in one continuous movement and take your hands back to your heels.

4 Keeping your hips forwards, take your head right back. Breathe normally through the stretch, lifting up through your thighs and pressing your feet into the floor. Hold the position for about 30 seconds and then come up.

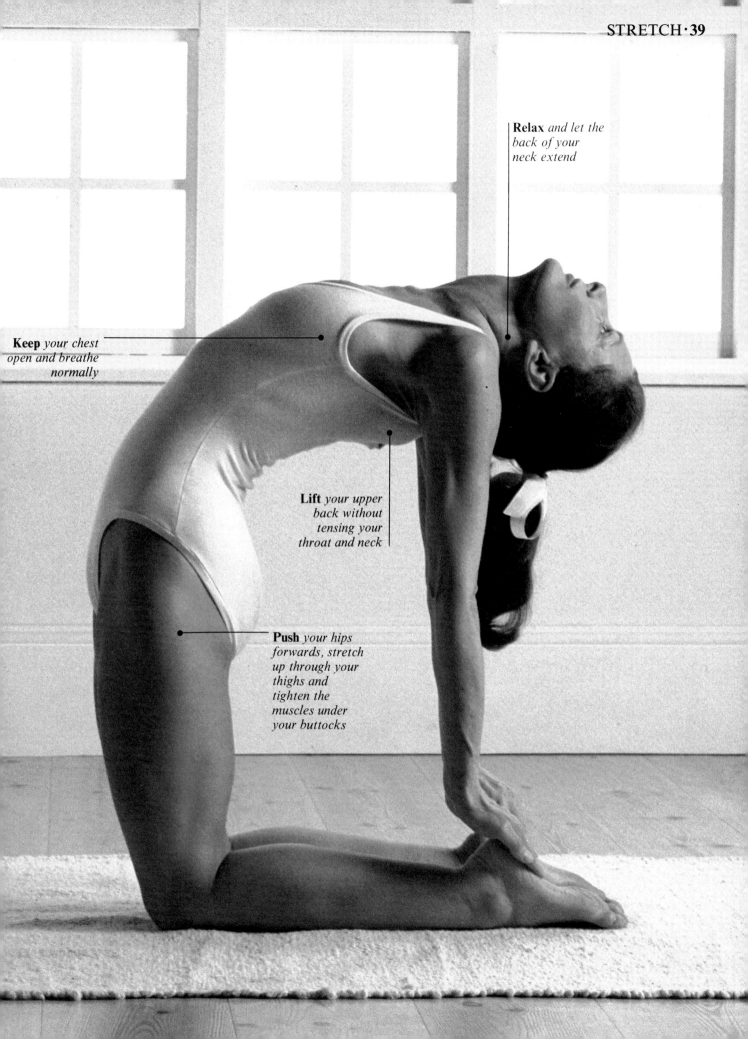

Relax *and let the back of your neck extend*

Keep *your chest open and breathe normally*

Lift *your upper back without tensing your throat and neck*

Push *your hips forwards, stretch up through your thighs and tighten the muscles under your buttocks*

·BACKWARDS·
LESS STRETCH

Before you attempt the basic position, you need to have strong back muscles and a good extension at the hips, otherwise you will feel constriction at the back of your waist. Do these stretches with your spine long and your chest open.

First stretch
Put a strong chair against the wall so that it cannot slip. You can also use the edge of a sofa or bed. Kneel down with your back to it. Sitting on your heels, bring your hands back and grasp the chair firmly. Push against it so that you lift up your hips away from your heels, tightening the muscles underneath your buttocks, and bring your shoulders back. Take your thighs as far forwards as possible. Lift your chest up from your hips, getting as much curve in your spine as you can. Lengthen your neck and keep looking forwards.

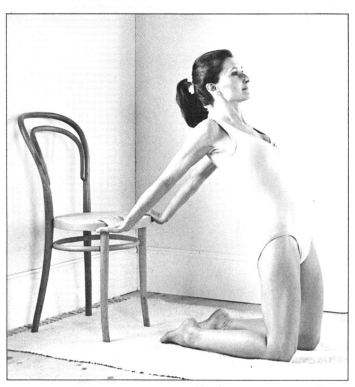

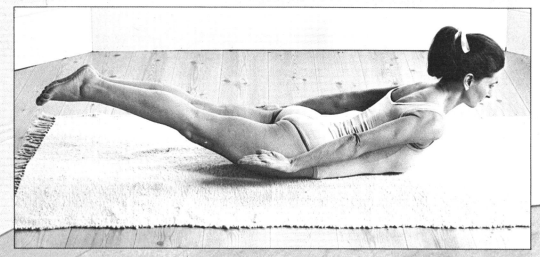

Second stretch
Lie on your front on a rug or blanket with your arms down by your side and the palms of your hands facing the ceiling. Stretch your legs back and tighten the muscles underneath your buttocks. Breathe out and lift your legs and shoulders off the floor, keeping your knees straight. The whole spine must stretch, so do not take your head higher than your feet. If your neck is stiff, extend the base of your skull away from your shoulders. Breathe normally for a few seconds, then lower your feet and head, and rest.

· BACKWARDS ·
MORE STRETCH

Pushing against the floor with your hands increases the intensity of this stretch, so do not attempt the positions on this page until you have toned your back muscles in the "less stretch" and basic positions.

First stretch

Lie on your front with the palms of your hands on each side of your chest, fingers pointing forwards. Tighten the muscles underneath your buttocks. Breathing out, push down with your hands and the tops of your feet, and lift your trunk and legs off the floor, extending your spine and straightening your arms. Your weight should be taken by your hands and the tops of your feet. Breathing normally, hold for a few seconds then come down.

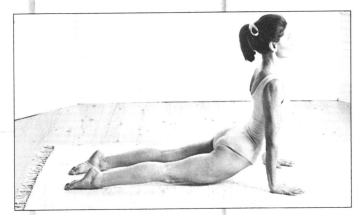

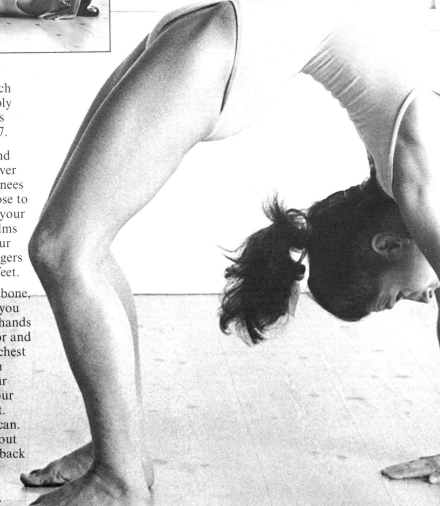

Second stretch

Don't attempt this stretch until you can comfortably do all the other stretches between pages 18 and 47.

1 Lie on your back and stretch your arms over your head. Bend your knees and bring your heels close to your buttocks, keeping your feet parallel. Put the palms of your hands under your shoulders, with your fingers pointing towards your feet.

2 Tucking in your tailbone, raise your hips. As you breathe out, push your hands and feet against the floor and come up, curving your chest as you do so. Straighten your arms and arch your back, without letting your feet and knees splay out. Come up as far as you can. Each time you breathe out stretch further into the back arch. Hold the position for a few breaths and then come down gently.

·UPSIDE DOWN·

The inverted positions are held for longer than the other stretches and provide a refreshing and revitalizing end to the practice session. They also promote mental relaxation. For the benefits to be appreciated fully your spine must be properly extended, so that your chest is open and breathing becomes smooth and easy.

When you start practising, stiffness in the upper back may prevent you from placing the weight high enough on the shoulders for the full spinal stretch. Only your shoulders, upper arms and the back of your head should touch the floor and there should be no undue pressure on your neck. Your chin should rest between your collarbones as the back of your neck stretches. If you feel that your head is crooked, come down in order to straighten it. Practice will gradually make the positions easier and the longer you hold them the more refreshed you will feel.

Caution: If you are menstruating or suffer from a specific medical condition, take medical advice before doing the upside down stretches. Instead you could finish the practice session by repeating the appropriate stretches on pages 26-9.

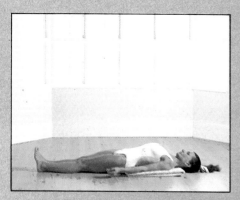

1 Lie face upwards with a folded blanket under your back. If you are a beginner or have stiff shoulders, you should put an extra thickness of blanket under your shoulders to protect your neck.

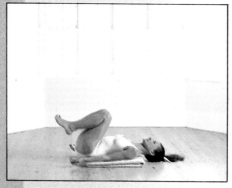

2 Press your hands against the floor. Keeping your shoulders down and your chest open, bend your knees and raise your legs over your waist. Take two or three deep breaths.

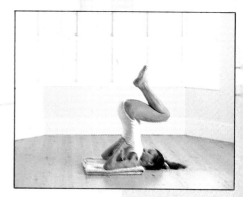

3 Pushing your palms against the floor, swing your knees up and over your head. You will feel the stretch in your upper back. Keep your arms close to your body, bend your elbows and support your back with your hands, your fingers spread horizontally.

Keep *your elbows close to each other* _____

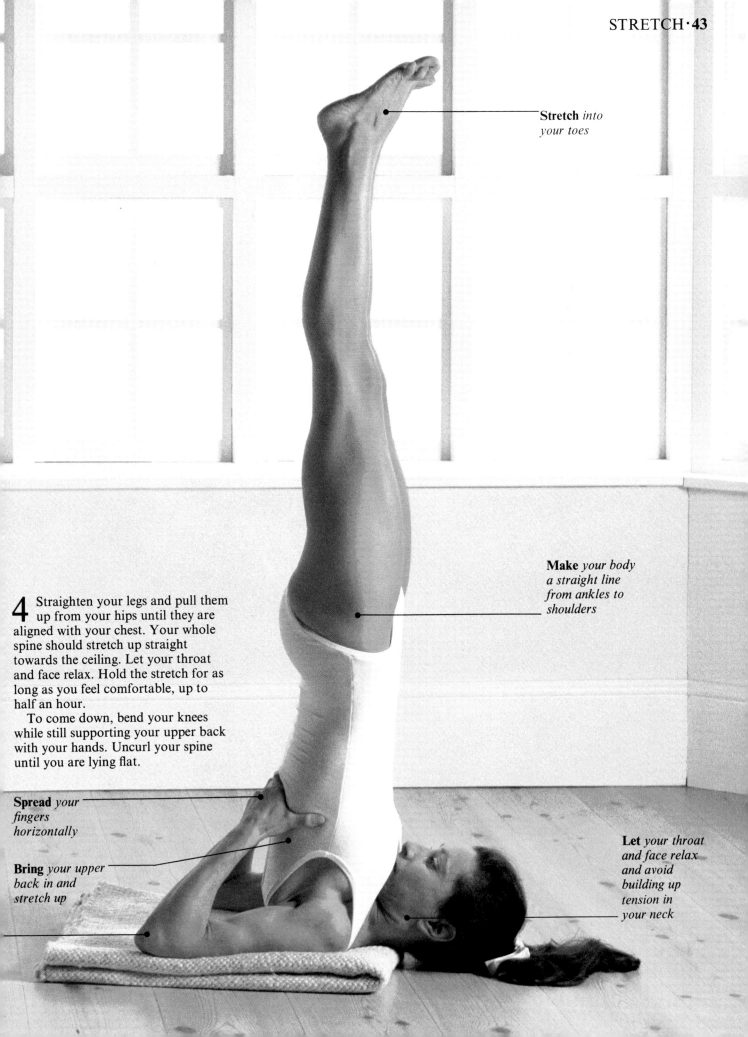

Stretch *into your toes*

Make *your body a straight line from ankles to shoulders*

4 Straighten your legs and pull them up from your hips until they are aligned with your chest. Your whole spine should stretch up straight towards the ceiling. Let your throat and face relax. Hold the stretch for as long as you feel comfortable, up to half an hour.

To come down, bend your knees while still supporting your upper back with your hands. Uncurl your spine until you are lying flat.

Spread *your fingers horizontally*

Bring *your upper back in and stretch up*

Let *your throat and face relax and avoid building up tension in your neck*

·UPSIDE DOWN·
LESS STRETCH

If you are very stiff or elderly you may find it difficult to swing your hips over your head in the basic position. This less demanding variation can be done with a chair, as shown here, or with your feet pushing against a wall. Make sure that you cannot slide as you push with your feet.

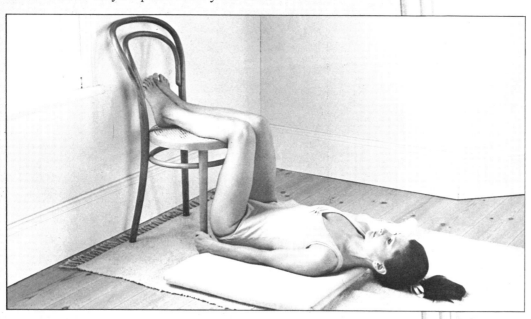

1 Place a chair against a wall. Lie on your back, a thick blanket under your shoulders, your knees bent and your legs comfortably supported on the chair. Hold on to the legs of the chair. Alternative position: You can omit the chair and adopt the same position with your hips lying close to the wall, your feet pushing against it and the palms of your hands flat on the ground.

2 Bring your feet along the seat of the chair and push against it with your feet, still holding on to the chair legs. Tighten your buttocks and slowly lift up your trunk.
Alternative position: Push your feet against the wall and support your upper back with your hands as you lift up your trunk.

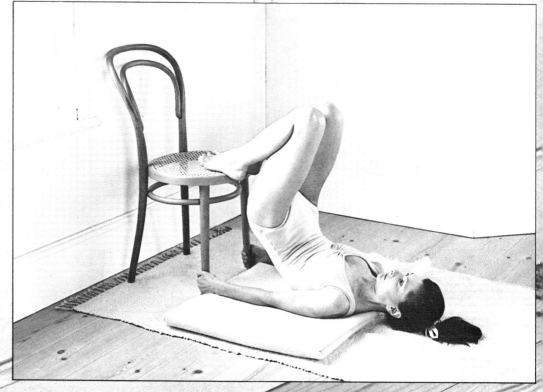

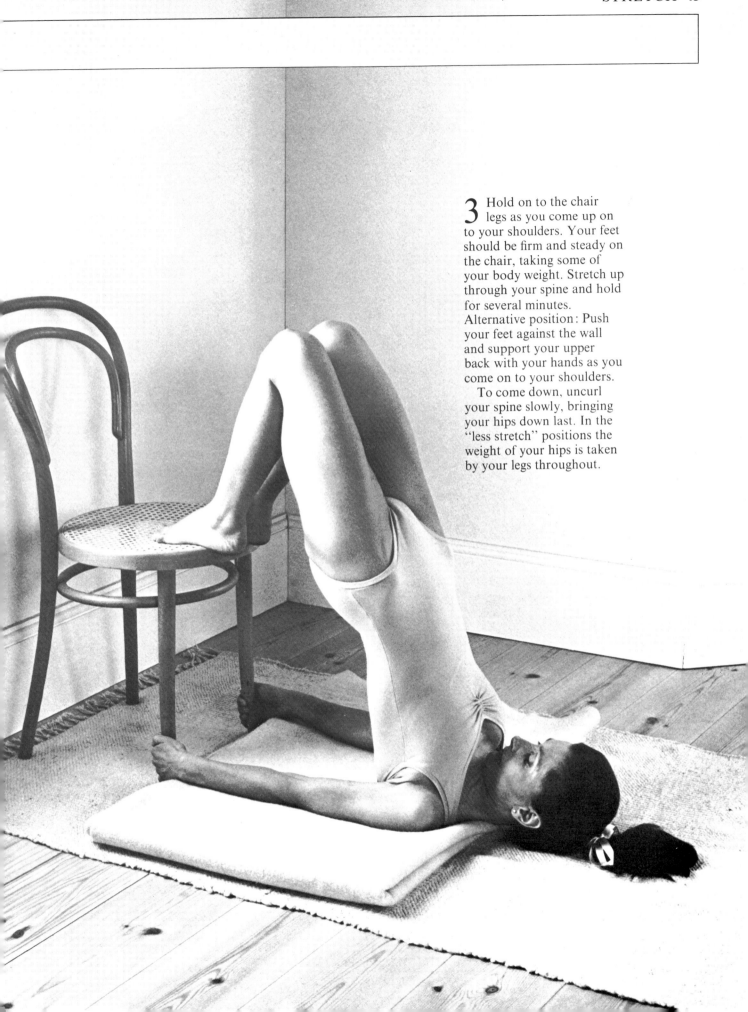

3 Hold on to the chair
legs as you come up on
to your shoulders. Your feet
should be firm and steady on
the chair, taking some of
your body weight. Stretch up
through your spine and hold
for several minutes.
Alternative position: Push
your feet against the wall
and support your upper
back with your hands as you
come on to your shoulders.
   To come down, uncurl
your spine slowly, bringing
your hips down last. In the
"less stretch" positions the
weight of your hips is taken
by your legs throughout.

·UPSIDE DOWN·
MORE STRETCH

If you find the basic position on pages 42-3 fairly straightforward, you can achieve a greater stretch by bringing your legs down over your head. Only go as far as you can while still stretching your back up. Make use of a chair or a stool if the stretch becomes too hard. The important thing is to feel relaxed and happy in the position, never to force yourself so far that you become uncomfortable. Use a good thick blanket under your shoulders to protect your neck.

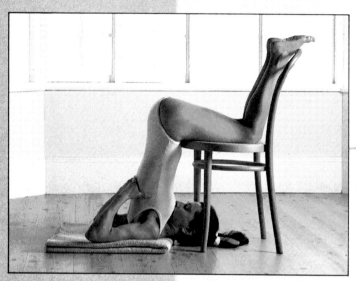

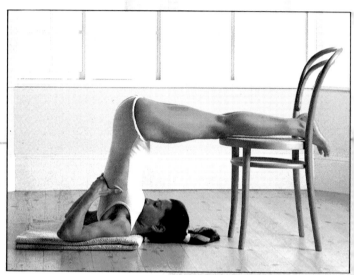

1 Lie flat on your back before bending your knees and raising them, first over your waist, then over your head, as in steps 1 to 3 on page 42. Rest your knees on the seat of a chair placed behind you. Support your back with your hands. Wait until you are comfortable in this position before trying the next.

2 Stretch your legs straight out along the chair so that they are at a right angle to your trunk. (It helps if you can get someone to move the chair back for you.) With the chair still supporting the weight of your legs, continue to lift up your spine while supporting your back with your hands.

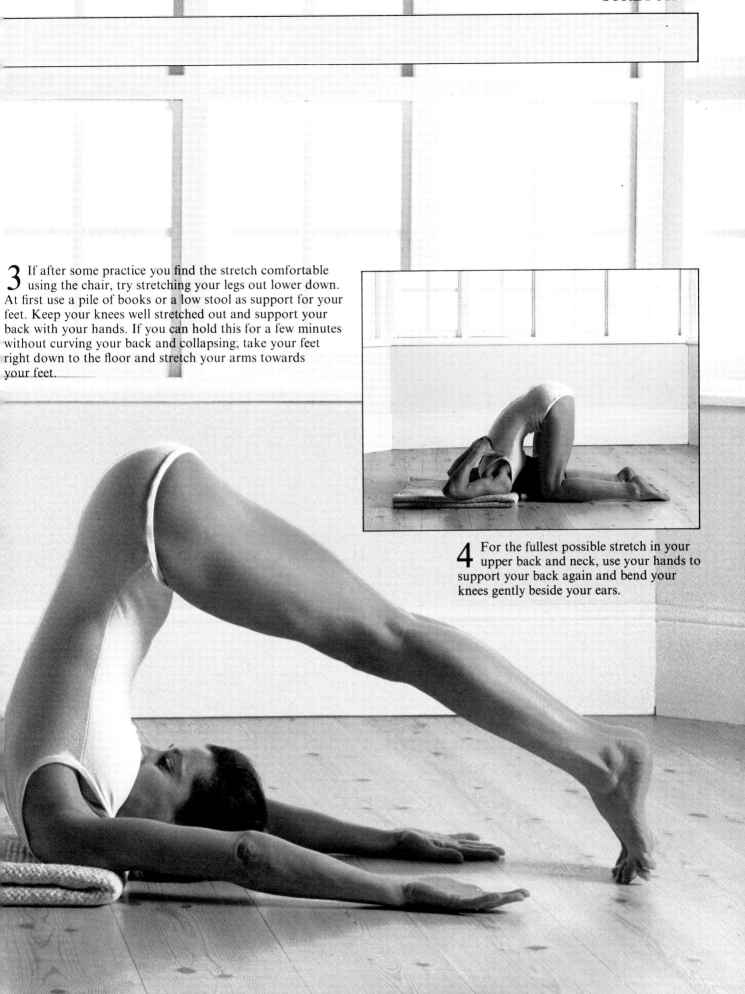

3 If after some practice you find the stretch comfortable using the chair, try stretching your legs out lower down. At first use a pile of books or a low stool as support for your feet. Keep your knees well stretched out and support your back with your hands. If you can hold this for a few minutes without curving your back and collapsing, take your feet right down to the floor and stretch your arms towards your feet.

4 For the fullest possible stretch in your upper back and neck, use your hands to support your back again and bend your knees gently beside your ears.

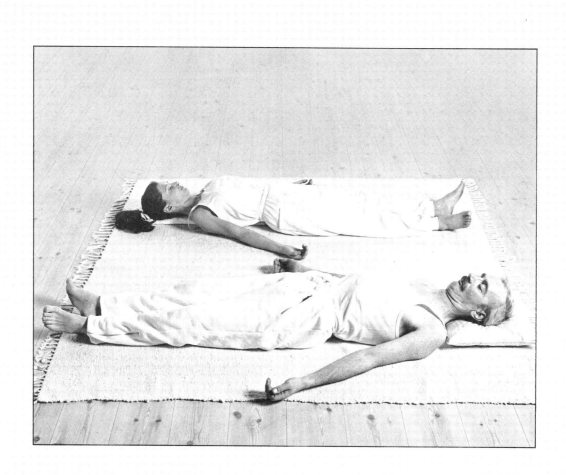

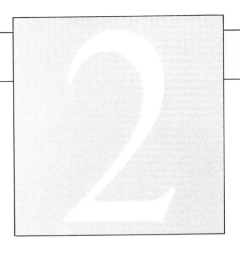

·RELAX·

The stress of day-to-day living depletes energy, as well as locking tensions into your body. Relaxation is a way of enabling you to follow phases of activity with periods of rest and tranquillity. It is not an escape from the pressures of modern life, but a chance to replenish spent energies. Far from being a luxury, it is an essential part of living.

For some people an absorbing hobby or sport provides a valuable form of recreation and a welcome antidote to the pressures of daily life; yet, while sports and hobbies can be helpful and relaxing, they can also open up fresh areas of tension. There are no substitutes for a brief daily period of total peace and quiet.

On a purely physical level, relaxation releases tension in the muscles. Your circulation improves, and your heart rate and blood pressure are regulated. But true relaxation goes further than this. Not only is there a release of tension in your body, there is also a calming effect on your mind as the rhythms of your brain change. This is not the same as going to sleep. When you begin to practise relaxation you may fall asleep, but being asleep does not necessarily mean that you are relaxed.

When you relax, you automatically breathe more slowly as your body needs less oxygen. This natural gentle rhythm can be a useful focus for your attention. The way in which you breathe is dictated by many things, including posture, tension and habit.

As your body becomes strong and flexible through stretching and your posture improves, the way you breathe can change. At first you should just let your breathing improve naturally.

After some months, when relaxation comes naturally and easily and your chest expands properly as you breathe in (see page 55), you can start to practise breathing slowly and more deeply. This will increase your intake of air without using up any unnecessary energy. Do not think of deep breathing as a discipline that you impose upon yourself, but rather as an extension of the relaxed state, achieved with no straining or effort. It should bring with it a feeling of refreshment and rejuvenation. If it feels difficult or strange when you first start, don't force it. Concentrate instead on improving your posture, stamina and flexibility in the stretches, and continue to practise the relaxation by itself until you feel ready to try again.

·HOW·TO·RELAX·

Learning to relax muscular tension is comparatively easy, but most people find it harder to unwind mentally. No matter how relaxed your body may feel, it is often hard to banish unwanted thoughts and worries and stop them flooding into your mind. The relaxation techniques here will help you relax mentally and physically. Do not be despondent if at first your mind continues to race; keep practising and you will find that you are able to relax and unwind more and more each day.

The ideal time to practise relaxation is after you have completed a daily stretch programme. Extending and flexing the spine and releasing tension in the joints and muscles will make you feel refreshed and able to let go. A further effect of stretching is to concentrate your attention on the movement of your body. As you focus on what you are doing you will acquire a feeling of wholeness, a feeling which should stay with you as you lie down to rest at the end of the practice session.

How you lie to relax is important. Your body must be evenly supported so that you do not tilt to one side as you let go and so set up a new pattern of tensions inhibiting deep relaxation. For this reason it is not suitable to lie curled up on one side or on your back with your head turned. The classic position for relaxation is shown opposite, while pages 52-3 suggest some suitable alternative positions for those who may find the basic one uncomfortable.

The basic position
The two stages of the classic position for relaxation are shown here. You start off with your knees bent and your feet flat on the floor (right), then you extend your legs one at a time without arching your back (above right).

Practising relaxation

Choose a warm quiet place away from bright light and take the phone off the hook. Remove any glasses or contact lenses. Spread a thick soft blanket on the floor and lie down on your back. Bend your knees and place your feet flat on the floor close to your buttocks. Let the back of your waist drop towards the floor and the strong muscles of your pelvis relax.

Without tensing your muscles, gently extend the curve at the back of your neck. Your chin will come down slightly, but your throat should stay relaxed. Let your eyes close.

As you breathe out, release tension in your shoulders by letting them drop down to the floor.

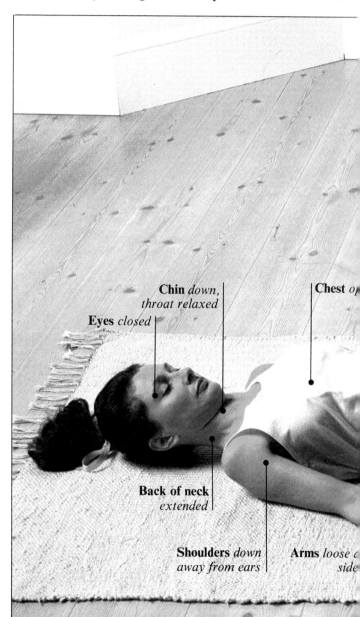

Chin *down, throat relaxed*

Chest *o*

Eyes *closed*

Back of neck *extended*

Shoulders *down away from ears*

Arms *loose a side*

Your arms will fall away from your body while the palms of your hands face the ceiling, your fingers curling naturally. As your shoulders relax, your chest expands horizontally, and there is a feeling of space, which helps your breathing. Try not to let your chest cave in.

Now extend your legs one by one, stretching them from your hips to your heels, and let your feet fall apart naturally. As you breathe out, let the weight of your body sink into the floor. Continue to breathe gently, allowing the quiet and stillness to permeate your whole body. This takes time to achieve, so be patient.

Concentrate on your face. Let your muscles relax so that the skin of your face feels smooth, especially across your forehead. Let your tongue rest behind your lower teeth, relax the corners of your mouth and keep your eyes closed. As your eyes become still your brain begins to relax.

As you breathe, pause for a second at the end of each out-breath, sinking your pelvis, your spine, your arms and the back of your head into the floor. This should seem a natural extension of your breathing. Let go of any residual breath and then allow the in-breath to come of its own accord. At first you will breathe consciously but after a time you will do it automatically. The gentle rhythm of breathing brings about deep relaxation: even at the end of a hectic day you will feel refreshed and revitalized.

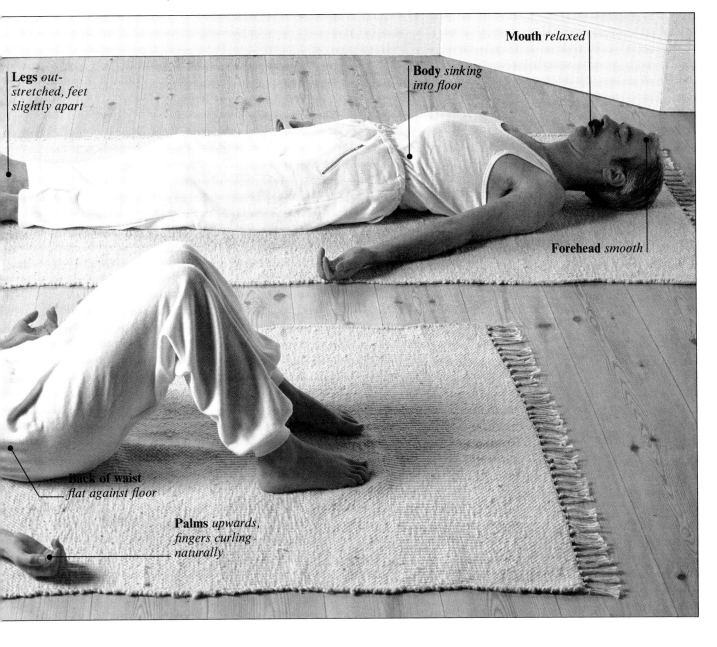

Legs *out-stretched, feet slightly apart*

Body *sinking into floor*

Mouth *relaxed*

Forehead *smooth*

Back of waist *flat against floor*

Palms *upwards, fingers curling naturally*

·ALTERNATIVE·POSITIONS·

If for some reason you find lying flat and still uncomfortable, then practise any of the alternative positions on these pages instead. The important thing is to practise relaxation daily after finishing the more dynamic stretches.

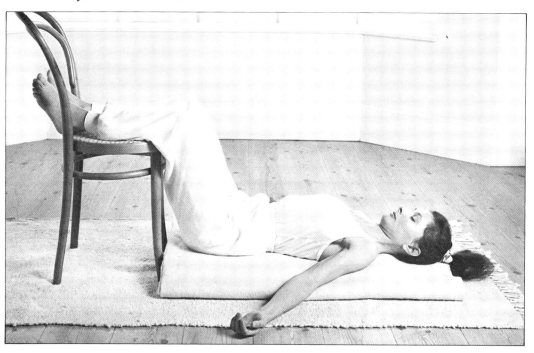

Easing a sway back
If you have a sway back (see p. 93), which arches up a lot when you lie down, you will find it hard to relax lying flat. Instead raise your legs and support your calves on the seat of a chair (if you have only a slight sway back, a cushion or rolled blanket under your knees may be enough to ease the tension at the back of your waist).

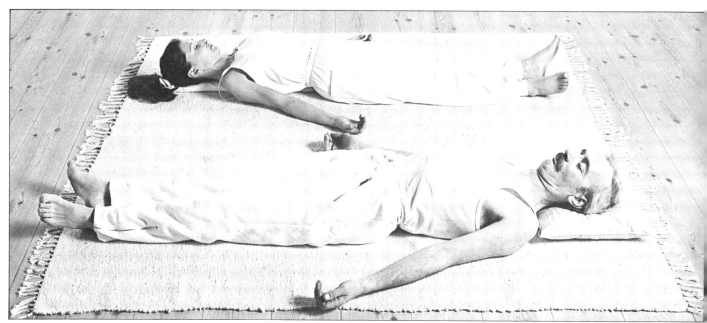

Easing stiff shoulders
If you find it difficult to relax your arms and shoulders, try lying with your spine resting on a tightly rolled blanket. This will help to release tension in your shoulders and open your chest. The roll should extend from the back of your hips to the back of your head and be narrow enough for your arms and shoulders to drop down towards the floor.

Easing a stiff neck and upper back
If your upper back is stiff and stooped the basic relaxation position is not suitable: your head will tilt back, the curve at the back of your neck will tighten and your chin will tip up too far. Instead allow your neck to extend freely by putting a pillow or two under your head. You should be able to relax your throat and jaw muscles.

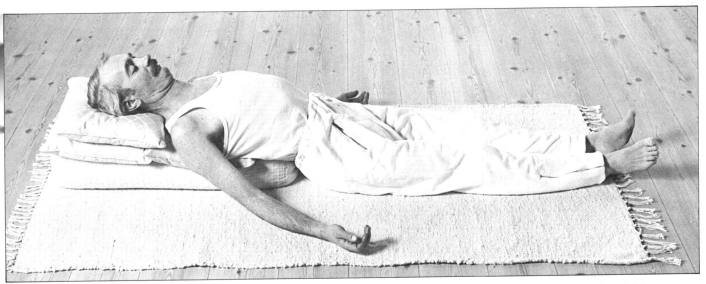

Easing breathing problems

Lying flat is not a good position for anyone with breathing problems. Instead use cushions to support the whole of your spine from the back of your pelvis to your head. Your arms should be free to extend away from your shoulders. Stretch them gently to release stiffness before you close your eyes.

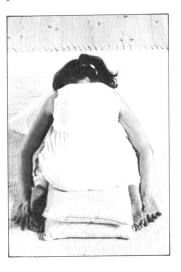

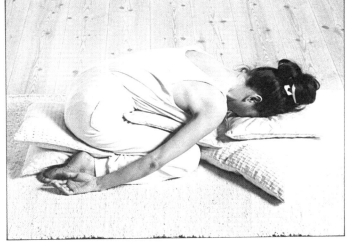

Kneeling forwards

If you do not feel at ease lying flat on your back, this position is ideal. Keeping your spine straight, kneel on a blanket and then stretch forwards onto cushions, letting your trunk relax. Support your buttocks either on your heels or on small cushions.

Sitting forwards

Try this position if you find that your mind stays active when you relax. Sit with your legs straight and together and put some cushions on top of them. Stretch out along the cushions, which should provide enough support to prevent your spine collapsing. The front of your body should feel extended and you should be able to breathe easily. Do *not* use this position if you have any back problems.

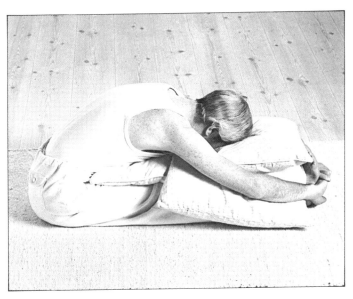

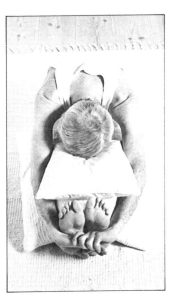

·DEEP·BREATHING·

Most of the time you probably pay little attention to the way you breathe. Perhaps you suddenly become aware of it during or after physical exercise – if you are breathing rhythmically while swimming, for instance, or if you are out of breath after running. You may not realize how your emotions also influence your breathing – you may sigh when depressed or hold your breath for a moment in anger. The reverse is also true: by concentrating on your breathing you can use it to influence your emotions.

Effective deep breathing
It takes patient practice to understand how to deepen your breathing while staying quiet and relaxed. Generally you take a deep breath because you need more oxygen and you use additional muscles to help you breathe. But this is stressful: just think of a runner gasping at the end of a race, forcing the muscles of his neck and shoulders to lift his ribcage. You should avoid straining and struggling with the muscles of the upper chest. Instead you should aim to increase the efficiency of your diaphragm and of the muscles that lie between your ribs.

Learning to breathe correctly
Lifelong habits, such as faulty posture, affect the way you breathe. The long muscle fibres at the back of your diaphragm extend well down your lumbar spine, and your diaphragm works most effectively when your spine is strong and flexible and correctly aligned. A body toned by stretching exercises will be fitter for deep breathing than one that is weak and poorly aligned. Other factors play a part in forming breathing patterns: tight clothes such as belts or bras restrict the movement of your body and can gradually alter the way you breathe.

You should check that you know how to breathe correctly before you start to practise deep breathing. This is as important as making sure your individual posture is correct before you start to stretch and exercise. If you lie flat with your hands on your abdomen, ribcage and chest as in the pictures opposite, you will be able to feel the correct movements. At first you should rest between each stage and breathe normally for a while, but eventually you will feel the entire movement in the course of one deep breath in. From then on you will no longer need to use your hands as a guide to the correct movement.

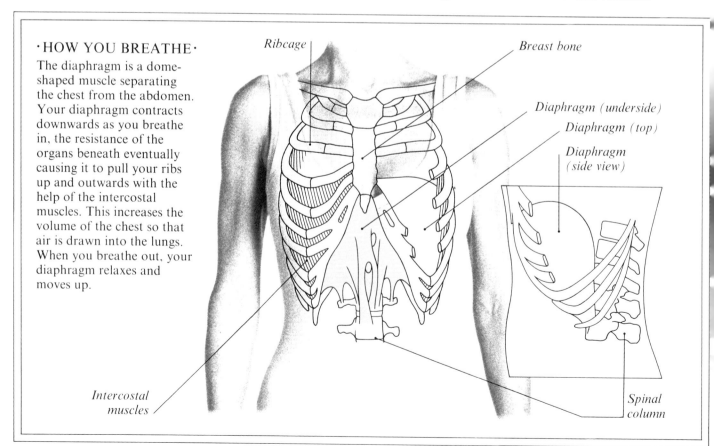

·HOW YOU BREATHE·
The diaphragm is a dome-shaped muscle separating the chest from the abdomen. Your diaphragm contracts downwards as you breathe in, the resistance of the organs beneath eventually causing it to pull your ribs up and outwards with the help of the intercostal muscles. This increases the volume of the chest so that air is drawn into the lungs. When you breathe out, your diaphragm relaxes and moves up.

Ribcage

Breast bone

Diaphragm (underside)

Diaphragm (top)

Diaphragm (side view)

Intercostal muscles

Spinal column

If you find it impossible to breathe correctly like this, stop trying to do any deep breathing for a while. Concentrate instead on the stretches and the relaxation. As you practise the stretches your body will gradually become flexible in every direction and you will tone your abdominal muscles. This will help correct a faulty breathing pattern. The lift from the lower abdomen and expansion of the chest in the "wide and strong" positions (see pages 22-5) are particularly effective.

Practising deep breathing

When you first start to practise deep breathing it is best if you lie down in one of the relaxation positions on pages 50-3. Wait for a few minutes until your body feels relaxed and you feel the quiet even rhythm of your breath. Start by breathing out, beyond the point where you would normally stop. Continue to release tension and let go as much of the remaining air in your lungs as you can, although this may seem very little at first. As you come to the end of the breath, pause for about a second so that you feel completely still and then breathe in slowly and deeply. Keep your face, tongue and throat relaxed as you do this, focusing your attention on the movement of the breath. Feel your ribcage gradually expand, the lower ribs opening first. When your upper ribs move a little at the end of the breath be sure to keep your neck and shoulders passive. Pause for a second and feel the back of your body resting on the floor. Breathing in should not have made you increase the curve at the back of your waist or neck and your spine should still be relaxed and supple, not hard or rigid. Then breathe out slowly as before.

To begin with it can be quite difficult to learn the right technique. If you breathe too slowly you may feel suffocated, so at first just try one breath out and in at a time, followed by a few ordinary breaths. If you feel like yawning, you need to breathe in a little more freely and increase the volume of breath more quickly. Each breath should be smooth and steady with no jerks, so that you are breathing in and out at the same rate from beginning to end. When you feel comfortable doing this, practise continuous deep breathing, establishing a regular pattern with in-breaths and out-breaths of even length. After you have finished you should always be still for a while before you get up; you should feel relaxed and fresh afterwards.

Breathing correctly

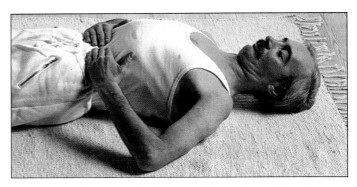

1 Lie down on your back on the floor and put the palms of your hands on your abdomen, your fingers pointing inwards. Your middle fingers should be by your navel. Breathe deeply and feel the movement of your abdominal wall beneath your hands. As you begin to breathe in, your abdomen should not push outwards or upwards against your hands, but should stay flat. Any movement should be slightly down, away from your thumbs and index fingers.

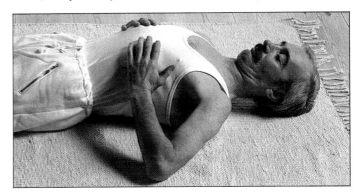

2 As you come to the middle of the deep breath in, put your hands on your lower ribs, with your fingers pointing inwards. This time you should feel your lower ribs opening out sideways and moving your hands apart.

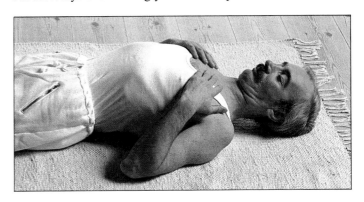

3 Carry on breathing deeply. Put your hands high on your upper chest, your fingers pointing inwards and your thumbs and index fingers just below your collar bones. Because the ribs here are fixed the movement will be less, but at the end of the deep breath in you should be able to feel a movement upward towards your hands.

·ALTERNATIVE·POSITIONS·

When you have mastered deep breathing while lying relaxed on the ground you can try it sitting upright. An upright position, with the spine aligned correctly in its four curves (see page 92), is in fact the ideal one. This is because when you lie down your diaphragm is slightly displaced and so your in-breath is less efficient. But sitting up straight without tension requires both strength and flexibility, and most people find it hard to hold the correct position for long at the beginning. It is very difficult to combine sitting up and breathing deeply and rhythmically with keeping your neck and shoulders completely relaxed and your spine stretching upwards. Trying to impose a pattern of deep breathing on a stiff tense body will only make you feel restless and disturbed, whereas deep even breathing should come as a natural extension of an already calm mind and relaxed body.

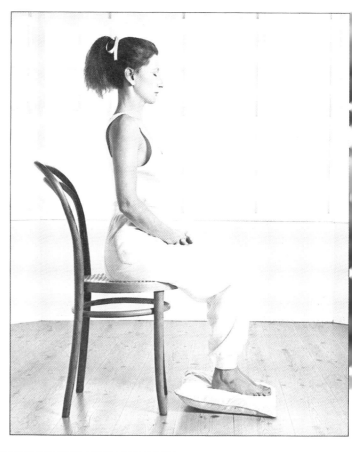

Sitting on a chair

The easiest way to sit with your spine aligned in its natural curves is to sit on a hard-backed chair with your feet and thighs comfortably supported and your back straight. Do not lean against the chair back but sit up tall and relax your shoulders. If the chair is too low sit on a cushion; if it is too high put a cushion or a book under your feet.

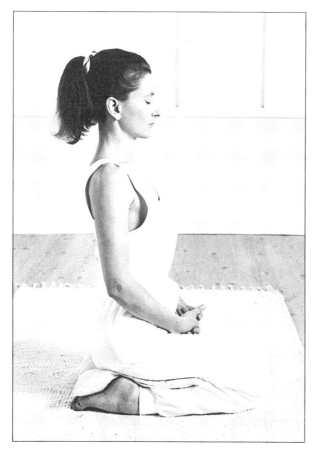

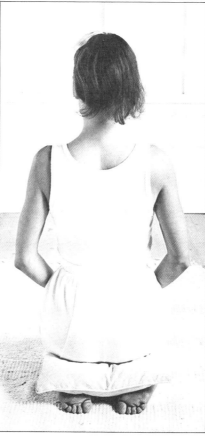

Sitting on your heels

This is a good position in which to keep your back erect and your shoulders relaxed. The problem is that if you sit like this for long you may get pins and needles in your feet. Try sitting with a folded blanket or cushion on your heels, taking care that your feet and knees are straight and the weight evenly distributed.

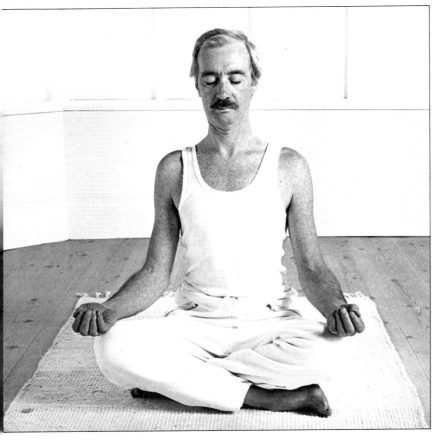

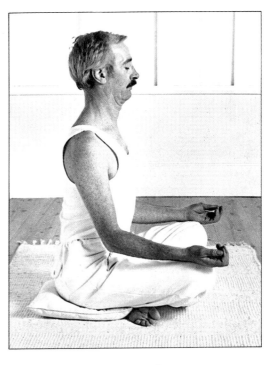

Sitting cross-legged on cushions
The position of your legs tends to push you backwards a little, so sit on as many cushions as it takes to raise your trunk comfortably, keeping your feet on the floor.

Sitting cross-legged
If you have flexible hip joints you can sit on the floor with your legs crossed. Your weight should be a little to the front of your buttock bones. You may find it hard to keep your shoulders relaxed with your hands on your knees (as above). It will depend on the length of your arms and the stretch and flexibility of your spine. You can put your hands wherever on your lap you feel most comfortable (right). If you use the cross-legged position, take care to alternate the way that you cross your legs.

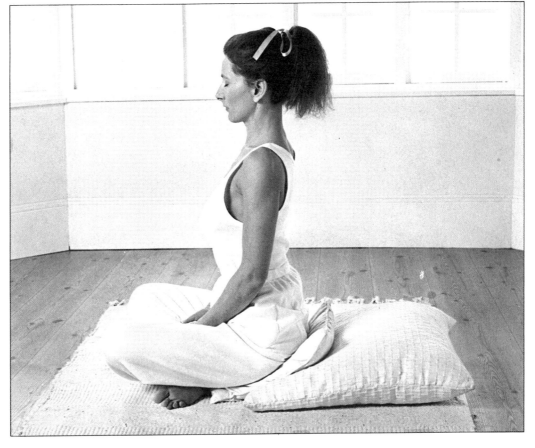

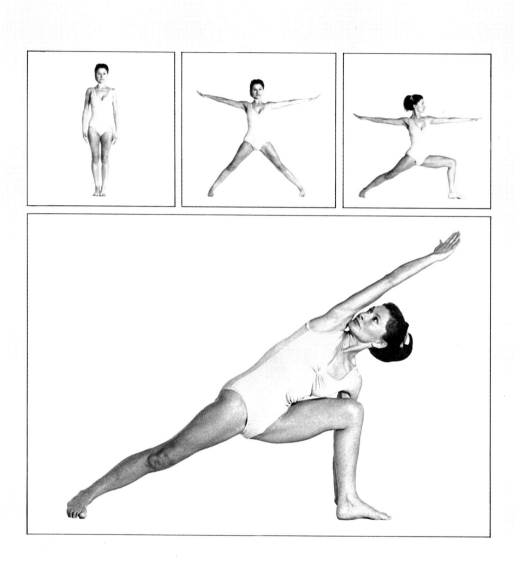

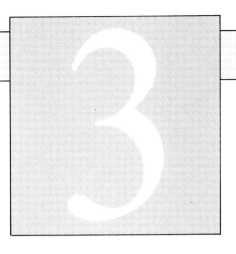

· STRETCH · PROGRAMMES ·

Methods of exercising which promise instant transformation are both suspect and dangerous. Change has to take place gradually: you cannot force your body to loosen up overnight. If you want to tone it up and make it fit and more supple, regular practice is essential. The ideal is a short daily session, but it is better to exercise a few times each week than to go all out for the occasional extended practice. It is also safer and more effective to practise for twenty minutes each day than to exert yourself frantically each week for a couple of hours.

Your daily practice must be planned and developed with care, for over a period of weeks and months your body will change. Because everybody is different, five programmes have been devised, each designed to last for about twenty minutes. The beginners' programme is ideal for those who have never done any stretch before; the basic programme should eventually be within the range of most people; the programme for the very stiff or elderly can be a practice in itself or merely serve for a few weeks as an introduction to the beginners' programme; the programme for the more supple is aimed at those who have practised the basic programme for some months and who feel the need to extend further; while the final programme is for those who are more experienced, who have practised for at least a year and who would like to give a little more time to daily practice.

You will get the most out of the daily programmes if you are already familiar with Chapter One; otherwise you will need to keep referring to the detailed instructions for each stretch. If for any reason you cannot do the upside down stretches at the end of each programme, finish by repeating the appropriate back to the centre position.

As you progress to more demanding programmes, give a little more time to the difficult positions, relaxing into them gently without straining. Remember also that stretch and relaxation go together; as you increase the stretch you should spend longer in the upside down position and take more time relaxing at the end of the practice, including some deep breathing while lying down.

The last two programmes on pages 70-3 are slightly different. They are relaxation programmes that last about an hour, to be practised perhaps once a month, on a day when you can give yourself a complete rest and stay quietly at home.

·BEGINNERS·

In this programme you learn how to feel the correct movement of the spine. You should practise it for some months before moving on to the basic programme. Those who are stiffer than average may find the programme on pages 64-5 more suitable for the first few weeks. To begin with, hold the stretches for a few seconds only, increasing the time as your body gets used to regular practice.

1 Straight
(p. 17)

Place weight evenly on both feet. Keep back long, shoulders relaxed. Stand straight, stretch up through spine. Hold for 1 minute.

2 Sideways
(p. 20)

Take feet 1m (3ft) apart, knees straight, arms out to side. Keep spine extended, chest open. Stretch sideways only, not forwards. Do not try to go down too far. Hold for 30 seconds each side.

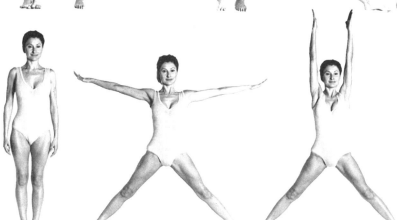

3 Wide and strong
(p. 24)

Take feet 1.3m (4½ft) apart, arms out to side. Stretch arms straight up above head. Keep back long, knees straight. Hold for a few seconds, stand straight. Repeat twice. Build up to holding for 30 seconds.

4 Back to the centre
(p. 28)

Kneel straight, sit on heels. Stretch arms up over head. Hold for 1 minute. Bend forwards, hips straight, arms by your side. Hold for 1 more minute.

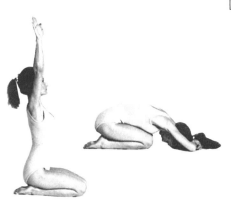

5 Forwards
(p. 32)

Sit up tall, legs straight out in front of you. Hold for 30 seconds. Bend forwards from hips, back straight, and catch toes with hands. Hold for 30 seconds.

Use a belt if you cannot reach your toes easily, or do forwards stretch shown on p. 65 instead.

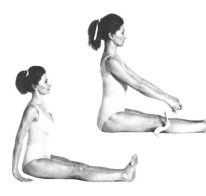

6 Twist
(p. 36)

Put chair so it cannot slip. Face chair, put one foot on chair seat, thigh parallel with floor. Twist around, stretch up. Open chest, relax shoulders. Hold for 30 seconds each side.

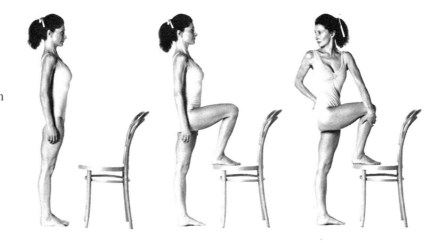

7 Backwards
(p. 40)

Lie on your front, arms at side. Lift legs and shoulders off floor. Lengthen spine, open chest, stretch back of neck. Do not take feet higher than head. Hold for a few seconds, repeat twice. Build up to holding for 30 seconds.

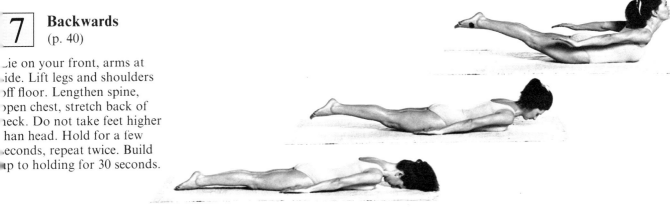

8 Upside down
(pp. 42-3, 46)

Lie on blanket. Press palms against floor, raise legs over waist, knees bent. Swing knees over head, straighten legs. Keep head straight, neck long, elbows in. Stretch up towards feet, lift from upper back. Hold for 3 minutes. Take legs back on to chair, keeping back long and stretching up. Rest knees on chair seat. Hold for 2 minutes.

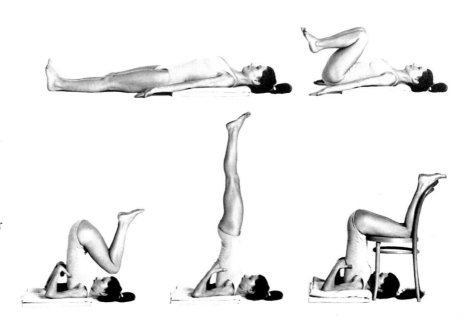

9 Relax
(pp. 50-3)

Lie evenly, head, spine, arms and hands well supported on cushions. Keep neck long. Stay in position for at least 5 minutes. If this is not comfortable, try one of the other positions on pp. 50-3.

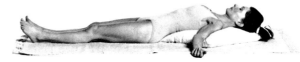

·BASIC·

This programme shows you how to put together in sequence the basic stretches. Initially practise the "beginners" programme on pages 60-1, but eventually the stretches here should be within the range of most people. Even if you are very flexible, practise this programme for several months before moving on to a more advanced one.

1   Straight
(p. 17)

Place weight evenly on both feet. Keep back long, shoulders relaxed. Stand straight, stretch up through spine. Hold for 1 minute.

2   Sideways
(pp. 18-19)

Take feet 1m (3ft) apart, knees straight, arms out to side. Keep spine extended, chest open. Stretch sideways only, not forwards. Hold for 30 seconds each side.

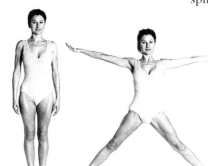
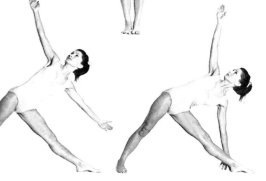

3   Wide and strong
(pp. 22-3)

Take feet 1.3m (4½ft) apart, arms out to side. Make thigh of bent leg parallel with floor, other leg straight. Hold for 30 seconds each side.

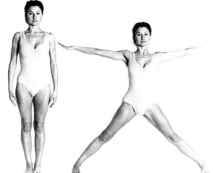
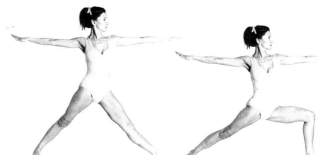

4   Back to the centre
(pp. 26-7)

Press one foot into other thigh. Keep standing leg straight, foot pointing forwards. Make back long, relax shoulders. Press hands evenly. Hold for 30 seconds each side.

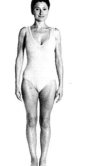
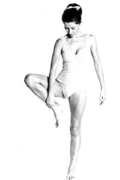
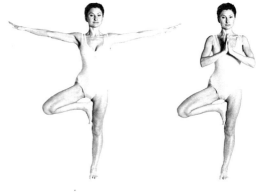

5   Forwards
(pp. 30-1)

Take legs very wide apart (1.5m or 5ft). Bend forwards, hips and head in line. Lengthen back. Hold with head up for 1 minute *or* hold for 30 seconds head up, 30 seconds head down.

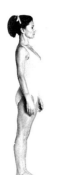
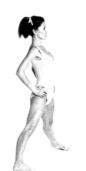
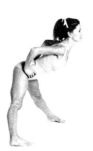
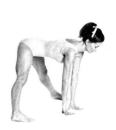

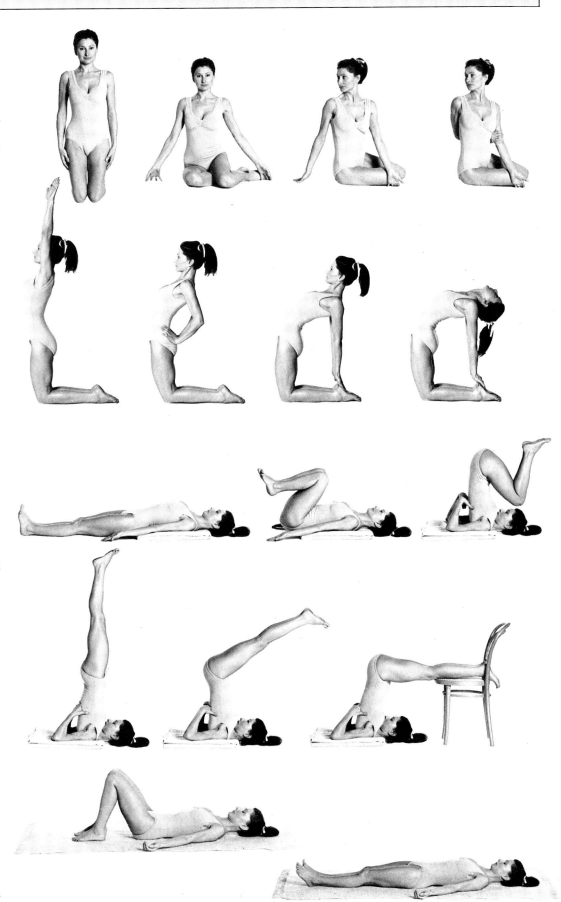

6 Twist
(pp. 34-5)

Kneel up, weight evenly on your knees. Sit back on heels, legs folded behind you. Stretch up as you turn, relax shoulders, open chest. Grasp arm behind back. Hold for 30 seconds each side.

7 Backwards
(pp. 38-9)

Kneel with knees and feet straight. Push forwards with hips. Lift spine, open chest and catch heels with hands. Extend neck, taking head back. Hold for up to 30 seconds.

8 Upside down
(pp. 42-3, 46)

Lie on blanket. Press palms against floor, raise legs over waist, knees bent. Swing knees over head, straighten legs. Keep head straight, neck long, elbows in. Stretch up towards feet, lift from upper back. Hold for 3 minutes.

Take legs back on to chair, keeping back long and stretching up. Have feet together, knees straight, legs resting on seat. Hold for 1 minute.

9 Relax
(pp. 50-1)

Lie with spine long, weight falling evenly on hips and shoulders. Keep head straight. Hold for 1 minute with knees bent and for at least 4 minutes, legs straight.

·LESS·SUPPLE·

You may want to practise this programme just for a few weeks before starting the programme for beginners on pages 60-1, but it has also been designed as a daily practice in itself for those who are elderly or particularly stiff. Gradually increase the length of time you hold each position. Remember not to hold your breath as you stretch, releasing gently into the positions without strain.

 Straight
(p. 17)

Place weight evenly on both feet. Keep back long, shoulders relaxed. Stand straight, stretch up through spine. Hold for 1 minute.

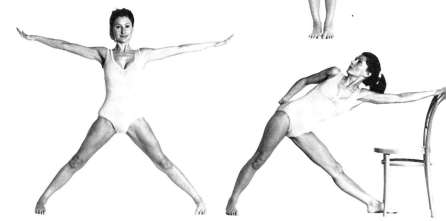

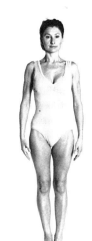 **Sideways**
(p. 20)

Take feet 1m (3ft) apart, arches lifted. Knees straight, stretch out as you reach sideways to chair. Look up, relax neck and shoulders. Hold for a few seconds, repeat twice each side.

 Wide and strong
(p. 24)

Take feet wide apart, legs straight, toes forwards. Release shoulders, stretch wide. Hold for a few seconds, stand straight. Repeat twice.

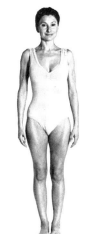
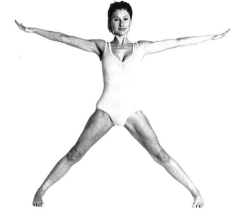

 Back to the centre
(p. 28)

Lie flat on your back, weight evenly distributed. Relax hips as you bend one leg. Keep other leg straight on floor, knee tight. Hold for 1 minute on each side.

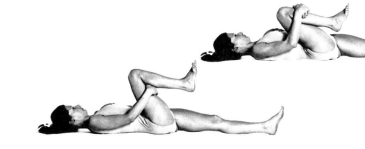

Forwards
(p. 32)

Stand straight, arms above head. Bend from hips, stretch towards chair, feet slightly apart, toes pointing forwards, knees straight. Lengthen back, relax shoulders. Hold for 30 seconds.

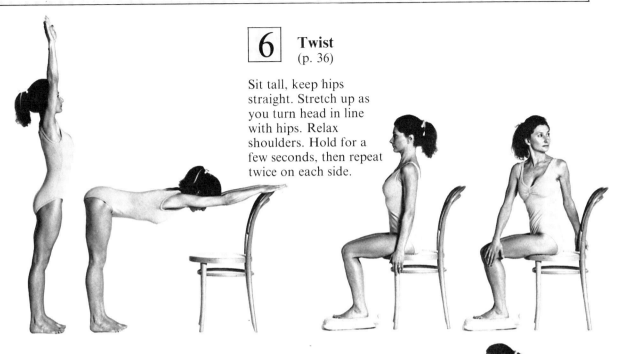

6 **Twist**
(p. 36)

Sit tall, keep hips straight. Stretch up as you turn head in line with hips. Relax shoulders. Hold for a few seconds, then repeat twice on each side.

 Backwards
(p. 40)

Put chair so it cannot slip. Kneel straight, push hips forwards. Lift up as you bend back. Hold for a few seconds, repeat twice.

 Upside down
(pp. 44-5)

Have blanket under shoulders and back. Hold chair so it cannot slip. Keep head straight. Press feet against chair seat, lift up from upper back. Hold for up to 2 minutes.

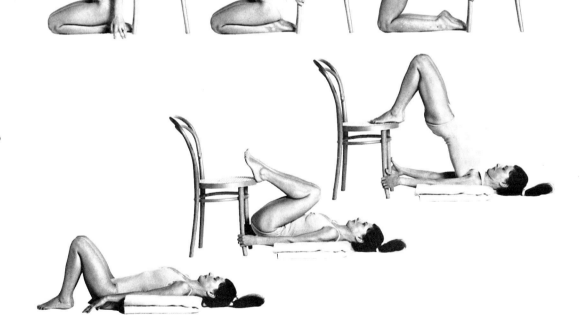

 Relax
(pp. 50-3)

Lie evenly, head, spine, arms and hands well supported on cushions. Keep neck long. Stay in position for at least 5 minutes. If this is not comfortable, try one of the other positions on pp. 50-3.

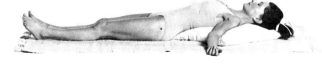

·MORE·SUPPLE·

If you are strong and supple, you may feel after some months of regular practice that you need to extend further in the stretches than the basic programme allows. If you like, you can practise this programme twice a week while carrying on with the basic programme on the other days.

1 Straight
(p. 17)

Place weight evenly on both feet. Keep back long, shoulders relaxed. Stand straight, stretch up through spine. Hold for 1 minute.

2 Sideways
(p. 21)

Take feet 1.3m (4½ft) apart, knees straight, arms out to side. Keep spine extended, chest open. Press outside of back foot against floor, make front thigh parallel with floor. Stretch diagonally to side, look up. Hold for 20 seconds each side.

3 Wide and strong
(p. 25)

Take feet 1.3m (4½ft) apart, stretch arms up above head. Turn whole body. Lower hips, make front thigh parallel with floor. Keep back leg straight. Open chest, stretch up. Hold for 20 seconds each side.

4 Back to the centre
(pp. 26-7)

Press one foot into other thigh. Keep standing leg straight, foot pointing forwards. Make back long, relax shoulders. Press hands evenly. Hold for 30 seconds on each side.

5 Forwards
(pp. 30-1)

Take legs very wide apart (1.5m or 5ft). Bend forwards, hips and head in line. Lengthen back. Take head right down, hands between feet, elbows bent. Hold for 1 minute.

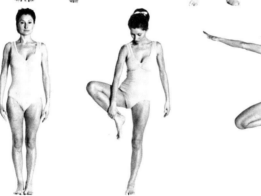
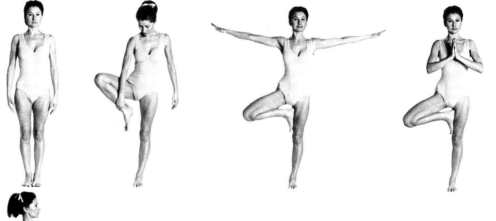
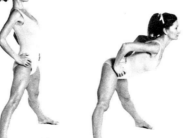
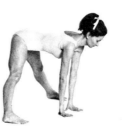
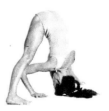

6 Twist
(p. 37)

Take feet 1m (3ft) apart, legs straight. Turn from hips, extend right arm over left foot. Make back long, open chest. Stretch top arm up, turn head. Hold for 20 seconds each side.

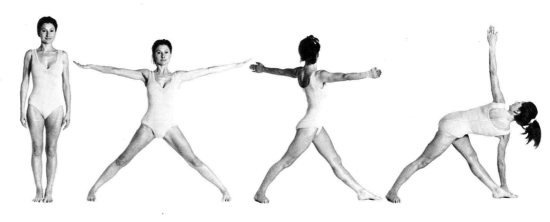

7 Backwards
(p. 41)

Lie on front, body straight. Lengthen spine. Lift up, arms straight, chest open. Extend neck, take head back. Take weight on hands and tops of feet only. Hold for 20 seconds, repeat twice.

8 Upside down
(pp. 42-3, 46-7)

Lie on blanket. Press palms against floor, raise legs over waist, knees bent. Swing knees over head, straighten legs. Keep head straight, neck long, elbows in. Stretch up towards feet, lift from upper back. Hold for 5 minutes.

Take legs back on to chair, pile of books or down to floor. Keep back long, stretch up. Have feet together, knees straight, arms supporting upper back. Hold for 3 minutes.

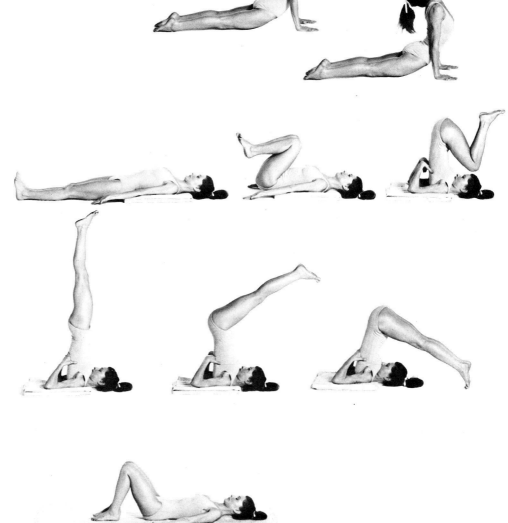

9 Relax
(pp. 50-1)

Lie with spine long, weight falling evenly on hips and shoulders. Keep head straight. Hold for 1 minute knees bent and 4 minutes legs straight. Introduce some deep breathing (pp. 54-5).

·ADVANCED·

This programme is suitable for people who have practised for a year or more, who have a good understanding of their bodies and who would like to give more time to extending their practice. Allowing for extra relaxation time, this programme will take about half an hour.

1 Straight
(p. 17)

Place weight evenly on both feet. Keep back long, shoulders relaxed. Stand straight, stretch up through spine. Hold for 1 minute.

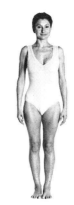

2 Sideways
(p. 21)

Take feet 1.3m (4.5ft) apart, knees straight, arms out to side. Keep spine extended, chest open. Press outside of back foot against floor, make front thigh parallel with floor. Stretch diagonally to the side, look up. Hold for 20 seconds each side.

3 Wide and strong
(p. 25)

Take feet 1.3m (4.5ft) apart, knees straight, arms up over head. Turn whole body. Lower hips, make front thigh parallel with floor. Keep back straight. Open chest, stretch up. Hold for up to 20 seconds.

Straighten standing leg, lift back leg, knee straight. Stretch out arms. Back foot and hands should be level. Hold for 20 seconds. Repeat sequence on other side.

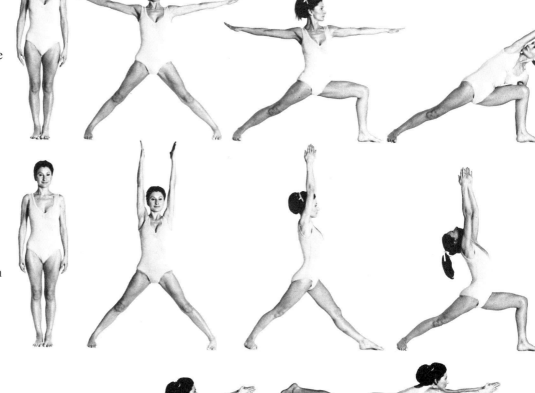

4 Back to the centre
(p. 29)

Sit on floor, legs straight. Spread legs very wide. Bend knees, bring soles of feet together. Let knees drop towards floor, lift up spine. Hold for 1 minute.

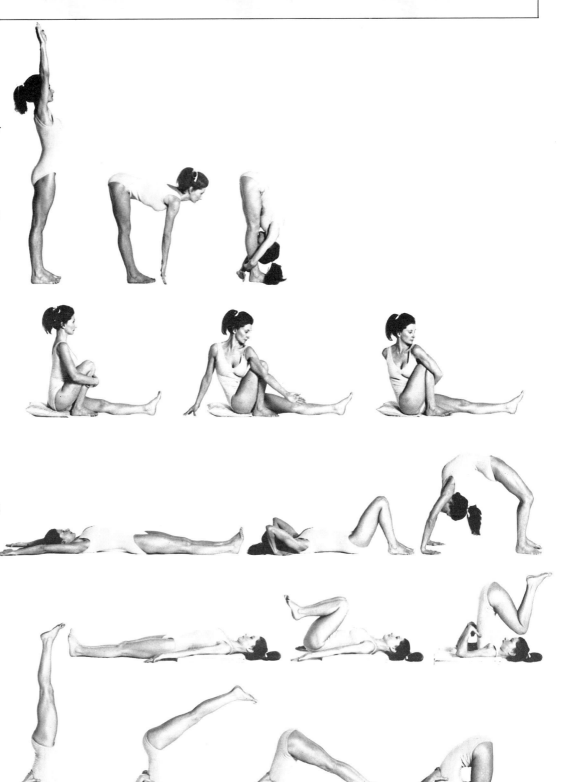

5 Forwards
(p. 33)

Stand with feet together, raise arms above head. Bend forwards, put fingers on floor next to toes, keep knees straight. Stretch forwards, head up. Hold for 1 minute. Bend down from hips, hold ankles with hands. *Don't force by pulling at feet.* Hold for 2 minutes (up to 5 minutes once a week).

6 Twist
(p. 37)

Sit with legs straight. Bend right leg, twist round. Take left arm round right knee, catch hands behind back. Hold for 20 seconds each side, repeat twice.

7 Backwards
(p. 41)

Lie on floor, stretch out, arms above head. Bend knees, bring heels close to hips, hands and feet pressing floor evenly. Raise hips, lift up trunk. Lengthen spine, open chest. Arch back, curve chest. Hold for 10 seconds, repeat twice.

8 Upside down
(pp. 42-3, 47)

Make body vertical, head straight, neck long, elbows in. Stretch up towards feet, lift from upper back. Hold for at least 7 minutes.

Take legs back down to floor. Hold with knees straight for 3 minutes. Bend knees close to head for final stretch. Hold for 2 minutes.

9 Relax
(pp. 50-1)

Lie with spine long, weight falling evenly on hips and shoulders. Keep head straight. Hold for 10 minutes. Do deep breathing at least three times a week, once a week in a sitting position (see pp. 54-7).

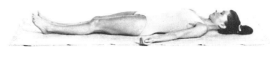

·RELAX·
LESS STRETCH

If you practise the "less supple" or "beginners" daily programme, you might like to try this more extended relaxation programme every now and then, perhaps once a month. The aim is to relax fully, not force or over-extend yourself. Breathe slowly and deeply as you hold the positions to release muscular tension as you stretch.

1 Straight
(p. 17)

Place weight evenly on both feet. Keep back long, shoulders relaxed. Stand straight, stretch up through spine. Hold for 2 minutes.

2 Up
(p. 32)

Take feet about 30cm (1ft) apart and parallel. Keep legs straight, stretch arms up above head. Breathe in as you take arms up, breathe out as you stretch tall. Hold for 2 minutes, breathing normally. Repeat twice.

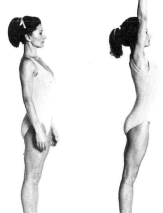

3 Forwards
(p. 32)

Bend from hips, feet slightly apart, toes pointing forwards, knees straight. Lengthen back, relax shoulders, open chest. Hold for 30 seconds.

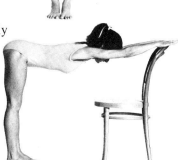

4 Forwards
(p. 32)

Take legs very wide apart (1.5m or 5ft). Breathe out, bend forwards, hips and head in line. Lengthen back, relax shoulders. Take head and hands down to chair seat. Hold for 30 seconds.

5 Upside down
(pp. 44-5)

Have blanket under shoulders and back. Hold chair so it cannot slip. Keep head straight. Press feet against chair seat, lift up from upper back. Hold for up to 2 minutes.

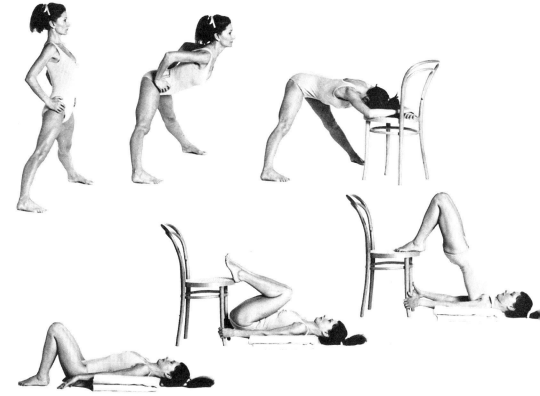

6 Flat
(p. 42)

Lie on floor. Stretch out, arms above head. Lengthen spine, particularly waist and neck. Hold for 2 minutes.

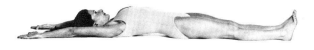

Upside down
(p. 46)

Have blanket under shoulders and back. Lie flat on floor, knees bent, heels close to buttocks. Lift up from upper back, come on to tops of shoulders. Take legs back on to chair, keeping back long and stretching up. Rest knees on chair, take arms down. Hold for up to 2 minutes.

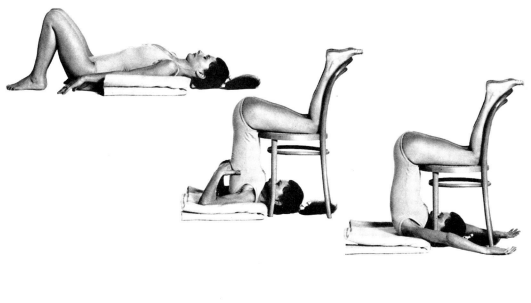

 Flat
(p. 42)

Lie on floor. Stretch out, arms above head. Lengthen spine, particularly waist and neck. Hold for 2 minutes.

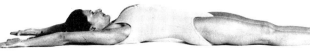

 Back to the centre
(p. 28)

Lie flat on your back, weight evenly distributed. Relax hips as you bend one leg. Keep other leg straight on floor, knee tight. Hold for 1 minute each side.

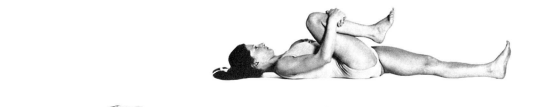

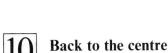 **Back to the centre**
(p. 28)

Kneel straight, sit on heels. Stretch arms up over head. Bend forwards, hips straight. Hold for 1 minute.

 Back to the centre
(p. 28)

Come up from previous position breathing in, stretch up. Breathe out, relax shoulders, stretch arms right up. Hold for 1 minute.

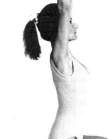

 Relax
(pp. 50-3)

Lie evenly, head, spine, arms and hands well supported on cushions. Stay in position for at least 10 minutes, then practise deep breathing for 5 minutes. Finish with further relaxation for 5 minutes more.

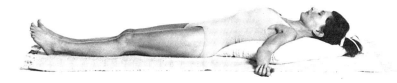

·RELAX·
MORE STRETCH

You can do this relaxation programme if you regularly practise the programmes for the more supple or experienced. It offers you the opportunity once a month or so to spend more time in the positions than in everyday practice. Breathe deeply as you relax into the stretches.

1 Straight
(p. 17)

Place weight evenly on both feet. Keep back long, shoulders relaxed. Stand straight, stretch up through spine. Hold for 2 minutes.

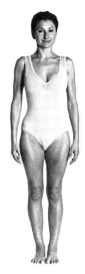

2 Up
(p. 32)

Stand with feet together. Keep legs straight, stretch arms up above head. Breathe in as you take arms up, breathe out as you stretch tall. Hold for 2 minutes, breathing normally. Repeat twice.

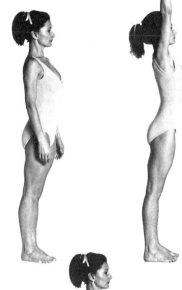

3 Forwards
(p. 33)

Bend forwards from hips. Keep knees straight. Stretch forwards, head up. Hold for 1 minute. Bend down from hips, relax trunk, let head drop as neck relaxes. Hold elbows, lengthen arms away from shoulders. Hold for 2 minutes.

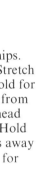

4 Forwards
(pp. 30-1)

Take legs very wide apart (1.5m or 5ft). Bend forwards, hips and head in line. Lengthen back. Take head right down, hands between feet, elbows bent. Hold for 1 minute.

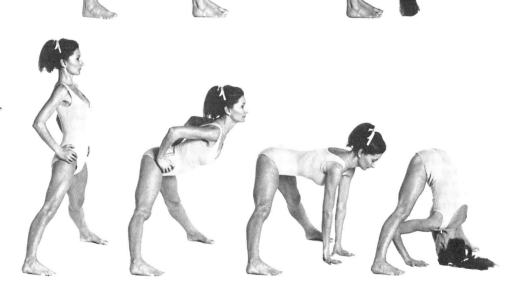

5 Upside down
(pp. 42-3, 46-7)

Lie on blanket. Press palms
against floor, raise legs over
waist, knees bent. Swing
knees over head, straighten
legs. Keep head straight,
neck long, elbows in. Stretch
up towards feet, lift from
upper back. Hold for at least
5 minutes, 10 minutes if you
are experienced.

Take legs back on to chair,
pile of books or down to
floor. Keep back long,
stretch up. Have feet
together, knees straight,
arms supporting upper back.
Hold for up to 5 minutes,
longer if you are experienced.

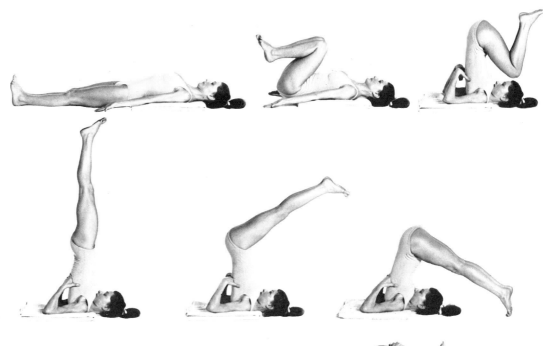

6 Back to the centre
(p. 28)

Lie flat on your back, weight
evenly distributed. Relax
hips as you bend one leg.
Keep other leg straight on
floor, knee tight. Hold for
1 minute each side.

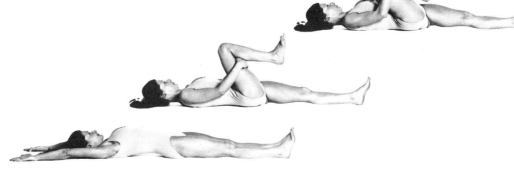

7 Back to the centre
(p. 28)

Kneel up, stretch arms up
over head. Hold for 1 minute.
Bend forwards, hips straight,
arms out in front of you.
Keep hips down, lengthen
back. Hold for 1 minute.

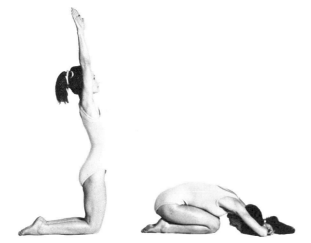

8 Relax
(pp. 50-1)

Lie with spine long, weight
falling evenly on hips and
shoulders. Keep head
straight. Stay in position for
10 minutes, then practise
deep breathing for 5 minutes.
Finish with relaxation for 5
minutes more.

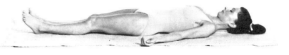

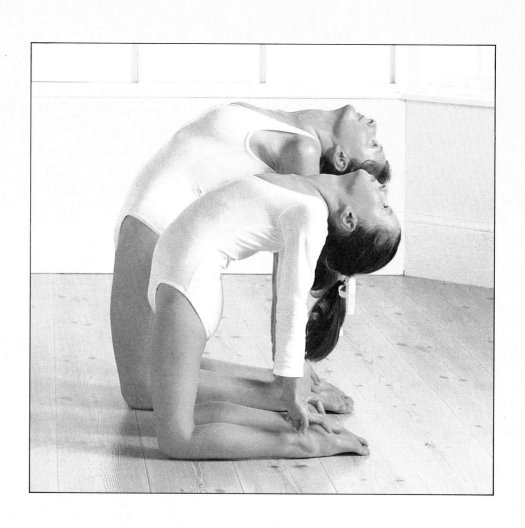

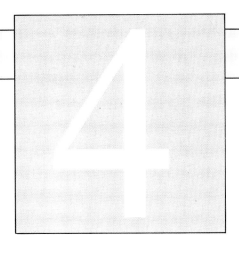

·STRETCH·TOGETHER·

Daily practice on your own is important, because you need to concentrate without distraction. But every now and then – perhaps once a week – stretching with friends or family is fun, especially with children.

When you stretch in a group, it is crucial that you know how to help each other properly. Before trying to help your family or friends, make sure you have a good understanding of the spine (see pages 92-3) and the basic stretches. Always refer to the full instructions in Chapter One for the stretch you are attempting. Follow those carefully and then try helping each other. The instructions in this chapter are directed at the helper.

It is very difficult to judge what is happening to your spine when you start to stretch. You can correct the front of your body by looking at yourself in a mirror, but to focus your awareness on the back of your body needs more skill. This is where another pair of eyes can really help. You can also take it in turns to use a pole or broom handle to align each other's spines. Pages 76-7 explain how the pole should touch the back and this applies to all the stretches where the pole is used in this chapter. The touch of the pole brings awareness to the back of the body: if the spine collapses and shortens, it will push against the pole immediately.

It is just as important to lie down and relax after practising with other people as it is on your own. You can take it in turns to read the instructions from Chapter Two to each other and you can make sure that your partner is lying straight.

Children do not have the concentration and stamina of adults, so do not make them too serious about the way they move. Encourage them to feel good about their own posture, to think tall when standing or sitting and not to slouch into chairs. Use the pole as you would for adults, but not for too long; adjust them quickly or they will get bored. They have more energy than adults and like to move much more quickly from one position to the next. Never force them, because their muscles and ligaments are weaker than an adult's. Let them stretch freely and naturally to keep their bodies mobile. It is good for children to relax for a few minutes afterwards, as they learn to appreciate a calm and quiet atmosphere. Although they enjoy relaxing with adults, don't expect them to stay quiet for as long – they do not have the patience.

·STRAIGHT·

Even those who feel they stand quite straight will find it helpful to have their posture checked with a pole from time to time. In a good standing position there should be a little gap between the pole and the back of your partner's body at the waist and at the back of the neck.

Checking correct posture (p. 17)

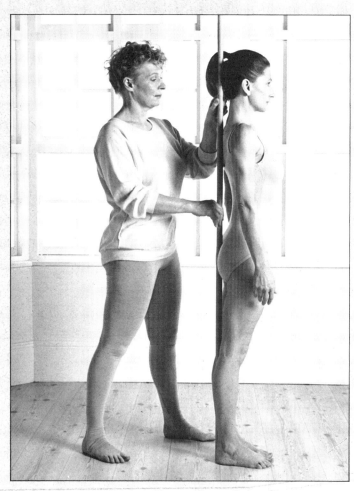

Identifying a sway back

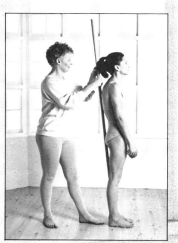

If your partner has a sway back, her upper spine will be very stiff and rounded. It will push the pole backwards out of line and tight back muscles will push her chin forwards. For more about this problem see the information about posture on pp. 92-5.

Overcorrecting a sway back

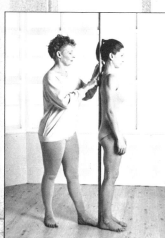

In trying to overcorrect a sway back, your partner may drag her lower back down and completely flatten her waist, so that there is no gap between the pole and the back of her waist. This is known as having a flat back. For more about this problem see pp. 92-5.

Let your partner find her natural position on her own as she stands up and stretches straight. Then place the pole vertically behind her, so that its base just touches the back of her heels. In the correct position the back of her head and her sacrum will touch the pole, which will also just brush the back of her chest.

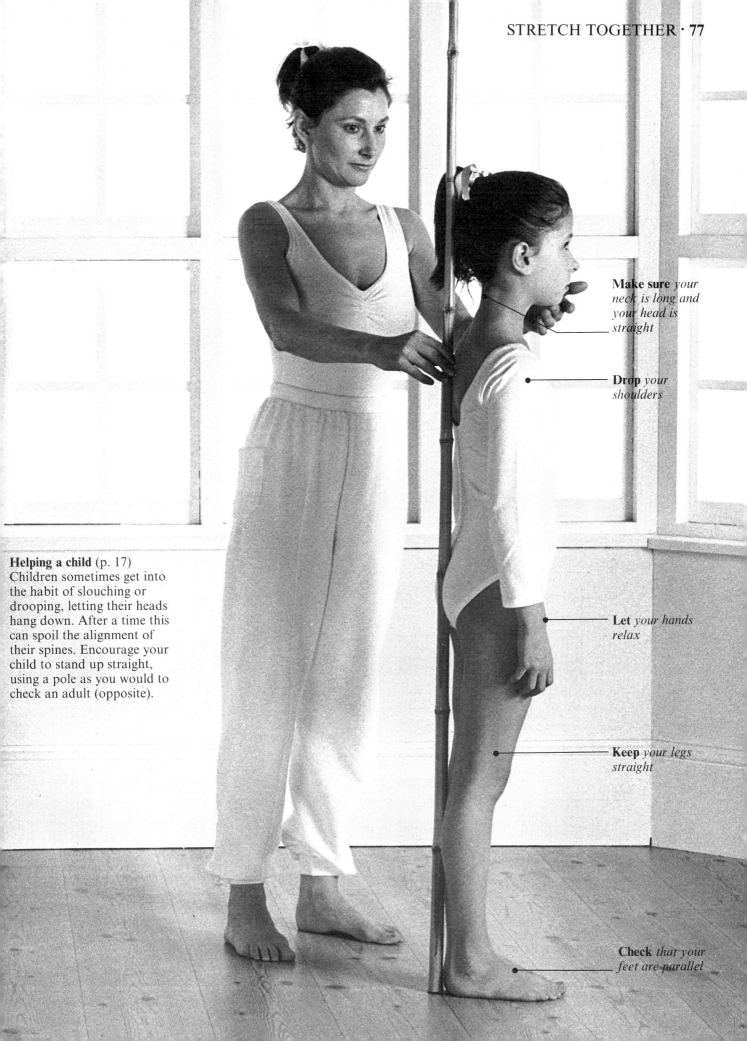

Make sure *your neck is long and your head is straight*

Drop *your shoulders*

Helping a child (p. 17)
Children sometimes get into the habit of slouching or drooping, letting their heads hang down. After a time this can spoil the alignment of their spines. Encourage your child to stand up straight, using a pole as you would to check an adult (opposite).

Let *your hands relax*

Keep *your legs straight*

Check *that your feet are parallel*

·SIDEWAYS·

When helping a partner to stretch sideways, line up a pole on her spine, as shown on page 76, before she starts to stretch to the side. As she moves into the stretch, re-align the pole so that again it lies along her spine, in line with her feet. You will be able to see at once if she goes out of line, and you will realize how important the "less stretch" positions are in achieving the right movement.

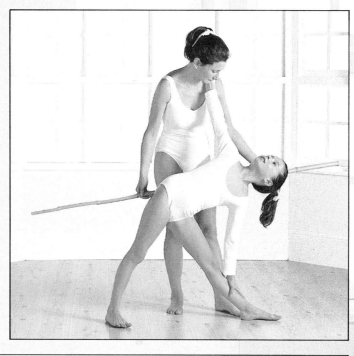

Helping a child (p. 20)
Encourage your child to stretch sideways, using a pole for guidance. Help her to open her chest and to stretch her top hand up. Don't make her hold the position for long, or she may become restless and lose interest in stretching.

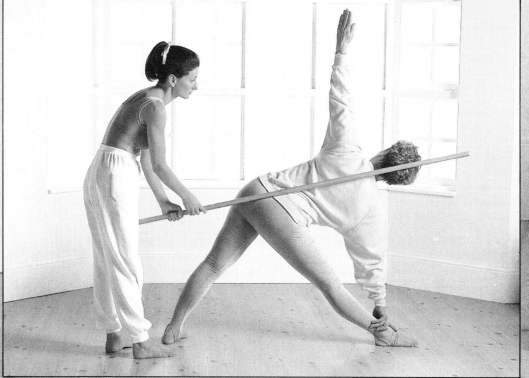

Basic and less stretch
(pp. 18-20)
Hold a pole against your partner's tailbone, following the line of her feet. As she moves sideways, do not let the pole swing backwards or forwards. It should touch her sacrum and the back of her head, leaving only a small gap at the back of her waist and the back of her neck.

Make sure *the outside of your foot stays on the floor*

More stretch (p. 21)

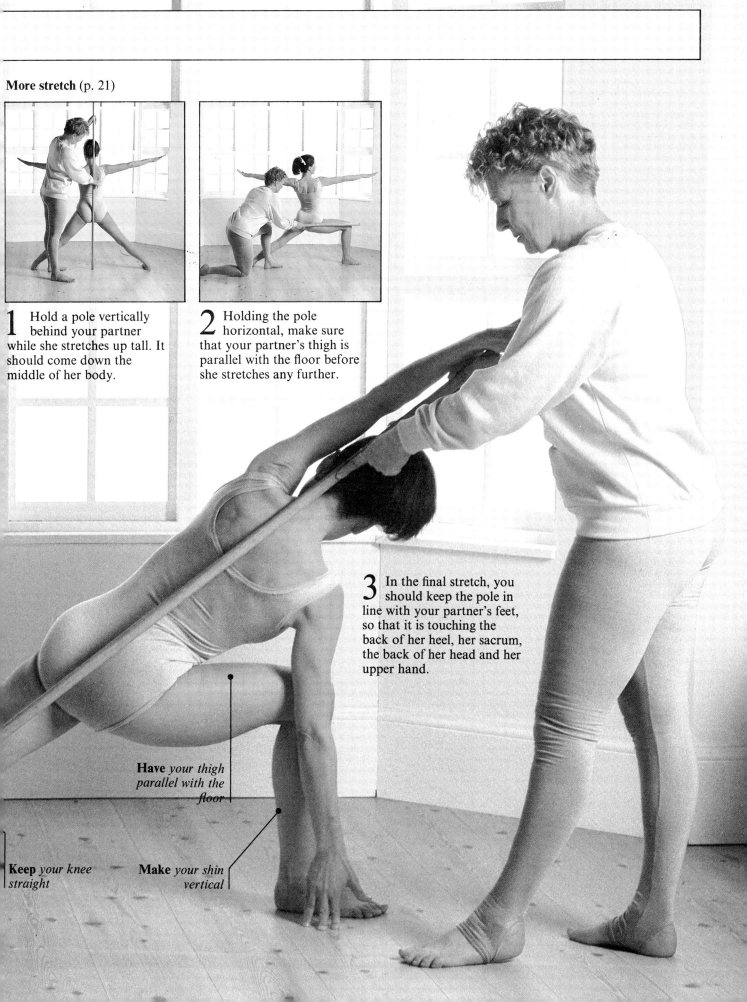

1 Hold a pole vertically behind your partner while she stretches up tall. It should come down the middle of her body.

2 Holding the pole horizontal, make sure that your partner's thigh is parallel with the floor before she stretches any further.

3 In the final stretch, you should keep the pole in line with your partner's feet, so that it is touching the back of her heel, her sacrum, the back of her head and her upper hand.

Have *your thigh parallel with the floor*

Keep *your knee straight*

Make *your shin vertical*

· WIDE & STRONG ·

Although all the wide and strong positions can be done with a partner, help is particularly useful with the balancing stretches. By offering a steadying hand, you can help your partner to concentrate on feeling the correct movement in the spine.

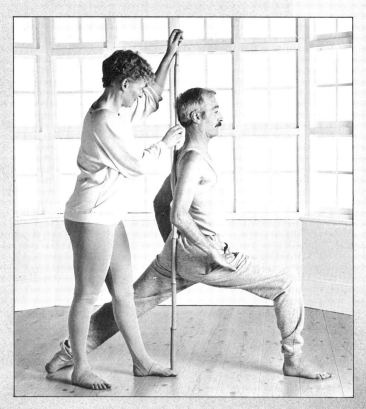

More stretch (p. 25)
Hold a pole vertically so that your partner is touching it with the bottom of his spine and the base of his skull. At first he should keep his hands on his hips, concentrating on feeling the correct stretch in his spine as he bends his front knee. Only when he can make a right angle at the knee should he take his arms up above his head.

Lift *your ba*
leg up with
knee straigh

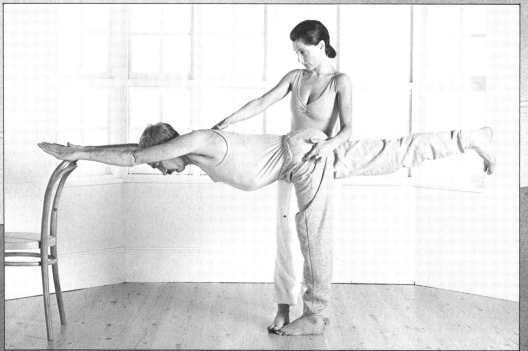

More stretch (p. 25)
Adults find this stretch difficult, because stiffness in the hips and shoulders and the fear of falling make it hard to stretch the spine fully while balancing on one leg. Get your partner to press his hands against the top of a chair. You can help to keep his hips level by extending back the hip of his standing leg. Check his alignment at the same time: his outer hip should be in line with his outer ankle and his shoulders should be at the same level as his hips. He should stretch horizontally from his pelvis.

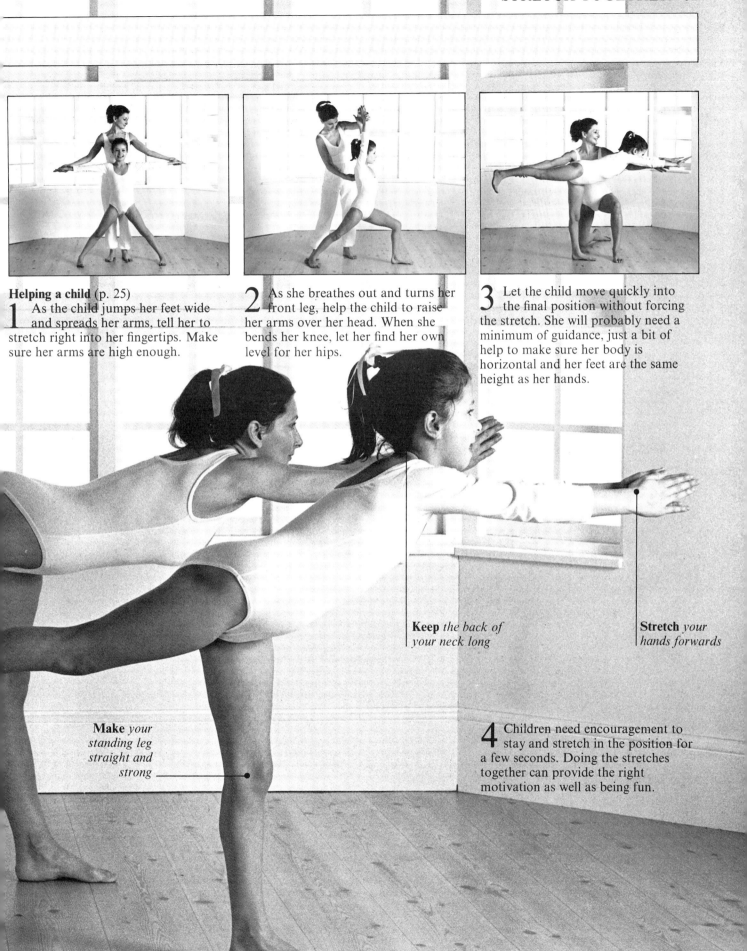

Helping a child (p. 25)

1 As the child jumps her feet wide and spreads her arms, tell her to stretch right into her fingertips. Make sure her arms are high enough.

2 As she breathes out and turns her front leg, help the child to raise her arms over her head. When she bends her knee, let her find her own level for her hips.

3 Let the child move quickly into the final position without forcing the stretch. She will probably need a minimum of guidance, just a bit of help to make sure her body is horizontal and her feet are the same height as her hands.

Keep *the back of your neck long*

Stretch *your hands forwards*

Make *your standing leg straight and strong*

4 Children need encouragement to stay and stretch in the position for a few seconds. Doing the stretches together can provide the right motivation as well as being fun.

· BACK · TO · THE · CENTRE ·

Applying gentle pressure to the thighs will greatly help your partner stretch in these positions. (Never press directly against the knee joints, as this can cause injury.) Your partner should not feel pain, you should merely be helping him or her relax into the stretch. When helping children, you should not use any pressure at all. Children can help adults, however, as long as they are careful and gentle.

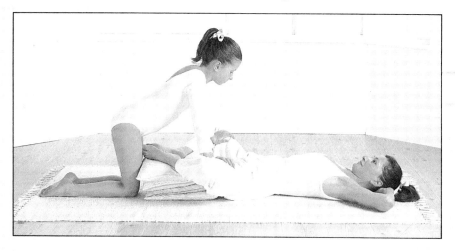

Hip stretch (p. 106)
Make sure that your partner is lying comfortably, her feet supported on cushions. Kneel down and apply gentle pressure to her thighs, rotating them outwards and pressing on both thighs evenly. If your partner is very stiff, use more cushions and make sure her feet are not too near her hips. This stretch is an easier alternative to the "more stretch" position (see p. 29).

Basic stretch (pp. 26-7)
Balance is a challenge to children as well as to adults, so enjoy yourselves doing this stretch together. Try to concentrate and hold the position for as long as you can. Because adults have stronger leg and spinal muscles, they can take their arms up above their head if they want an extra stretch; a child would find this hard.

Less stretch (p. 28)
A child who is light can safely stretch over an adult in this position, as long as the child's feet remain on the floor. The adult benefits because the extra pressure applied keeps her buttocks down on her heels. She can then extend her spine and move forwards more easily. Caution: Two adults should not help each other in this way.

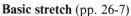

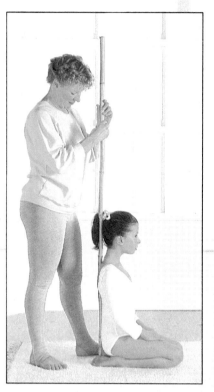

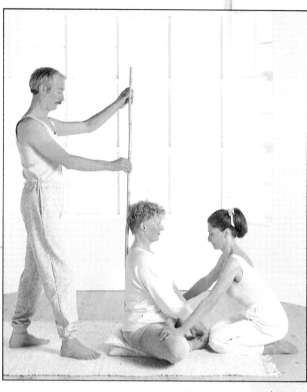

Less stretch (p. 28)
When your partner is sitting on her heels, hold a pole vertically against her back to check that she is stretching up properly. Make sure that her hips and feet are evenly placed and that her pelvis is not tilted. Then take away the pole so that she is able to bend forwards.

More stretch (p. 29)
Help your partner by gently extending her hips outwards, using only the minimum pressure needed to encourage the muscles to relax. Put your hands on her thighs, never on her knees. You can also help by using a pole.

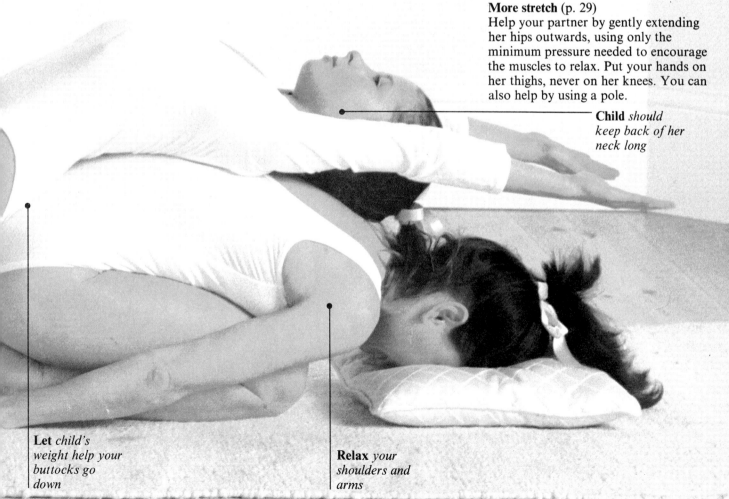

Child *should keep back of her neck long*

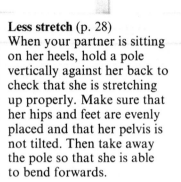

Let *child's weight help your buttocks go down*

Relax *your shoulders and arms*

· FORWARDS ·

Many people find the movement from the hips difficult in the forward stretches, as tight back thigh muscles (hamstrings) limit the rotation of the pelvis and place extra strain on the lumbar spine. By using a pole for guidance, you will help your partner to understand the correct movement more easily and quickly.

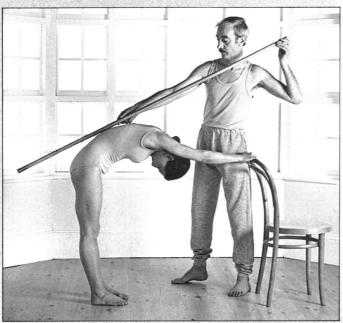

Less stretch (p. 32)
Help your partner by placing a pole behind her as she bends forwards to touch a chair. To begin with she may curve her back as she bends, pushing the pole away from her sacrum and head (left).

In the correct stretch your partner's spine should be parallel with the floor (below), with the pole horizontal. For this to happen, the backs of her thighs must extend, allowing her pelvis to rotate forwards and her lower spine to stretch out from her hips. Her legs should stay straight and vertical throughout.

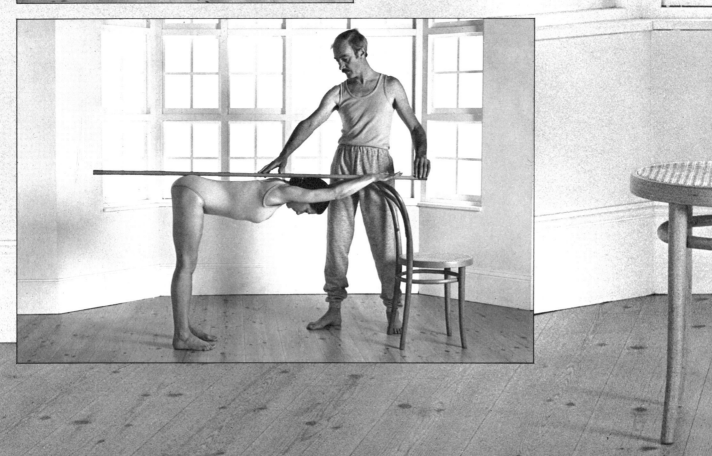

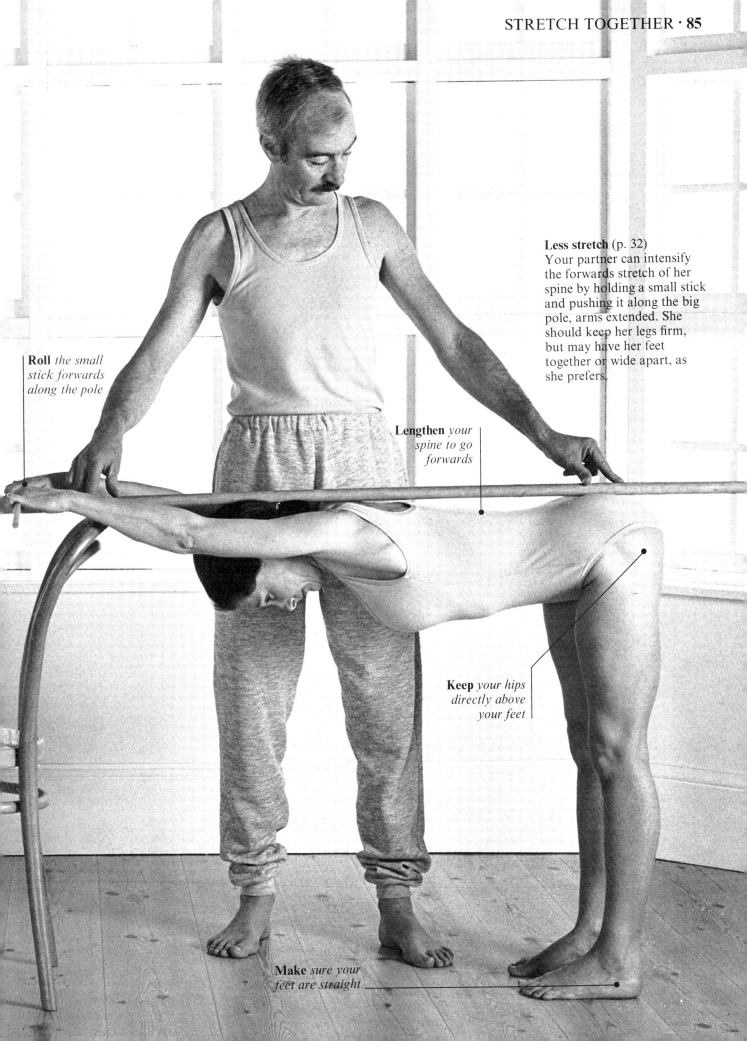

Less stretch (p. 32)
Your partner can intensify the forwards stretch of her spine by holding a small stick and pushing it along the big pole, arms extended. She should keep her legs firm, but may have her feet together or wide apart, as she prefers.

Roll *the small stick forwards along the pole*

Lengthen *your spine to go forwards*

Keep *your hips directly above your feet*

Make *sure your feet are straight*

· TWIST ·

You can help your partner to feel the correct stretch in the twisting movements by using a pole for guidance. Other possible ways of increasing his or her stretch are shown below; choose whichever ones seem appropriate.

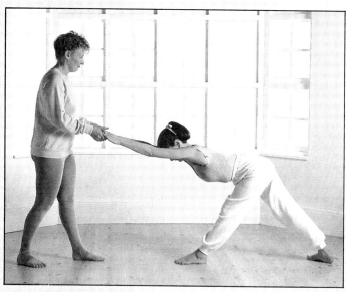

Extending forwards (p. 37)
You could help your partner extend her spine as she prepares to turn by gently stretching her forwards. Hold her hands high enough for her to move her lower back in.

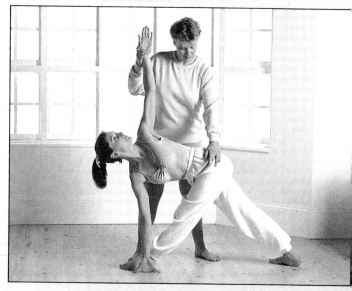

Extending her arm (p. 37)
While your partner twists, you could hold her upper hand and gently extend her arm upwards. This will help her turn her upper spine. Your hand on her hip will assist balance.

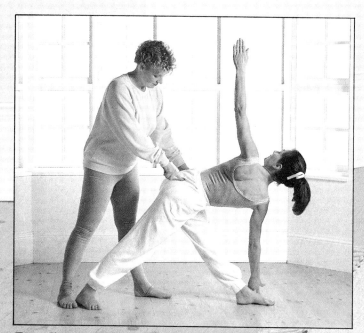

Extending her hips (p. 37)
As your spartner turns to the left, try gently extending her left hip backwards to help her twist more effectively. Her lower back should move in.

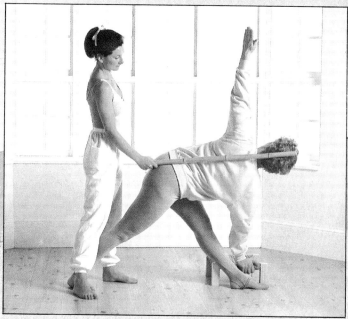

Using the pole (p. 37)
You could hold a pole behind your partner to help her feel the correct stretch. If she finds it difficult to turn properly, let her rest her hand on a stool instead of the floor.

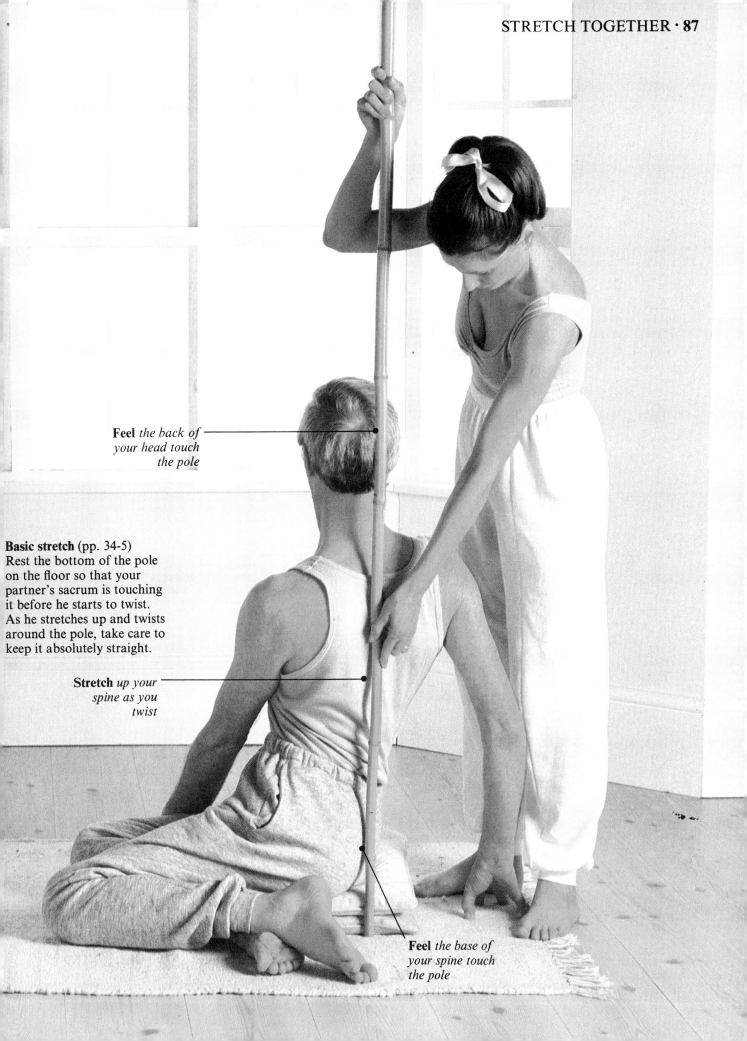

Feel *the back of your head touch the pole*

Basic stretch (pp. 34-5)
Rest the bottom of the pole on the floor so that your partner's sacrum is touching it before he starts to twist. As he stretches up and twists around the pole, take care to keep it absolutely straight.

Stretch *up your spine as you twist*

Feel *the base of your spine touch the pole*

· BACKWARDS ·

These stretches should extend the whole spine, not just the back of the waist. Helping someone in these movements makes it easier for him or her to stretch the spine while bending back. This is especially useful for a stiff person.

Less and basic stretch (pp. 38-40)
The stiffer your partner is, the more she will benefit from help. Pull her hips gently (far right), encouraging her to stretch from her lower back. Alternatively, loop a belt round her bottom near the tops of her thighs (right). Do not hold her rigidly, but give her whatever support she needs to achieve a good stretch with confidence.

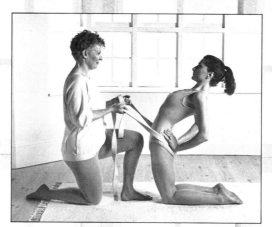
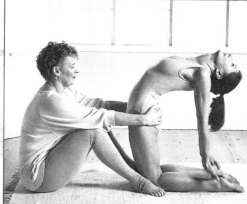

Less stretch (p. 40)
It's good if there can be two of you to help with this. First ask your partner to lie on his front and hold the other helper's knees (or a piece of heavy furniture, if there is only one helper). Then take hold of his heels and gently pull back so that, as he bends backwards, he can stretch against the resistance you offer. Do not pull his feet up too high.

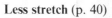

Stretch *the back of your neck*

Lengthen *the back of your waist*

Partner *should gently extend your leg*

· UPSIDE · DOWN ·

In these stretches the upper back has to lift up so that there is no pressure on the neck. If your partner's head needs adjusting, she should come down out of the position to straighten it.

Caution:
Never lift or pull people when they are upside down.

Basic stretch (pp. 42-3)

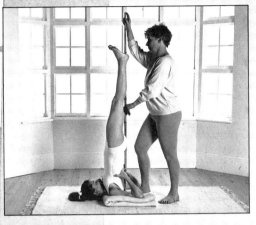

Encourage your partner to lift up her spine against a pole. If she becomes red in the face, she should do the "less stretch" pose.

More stretch (pp. 46-7)

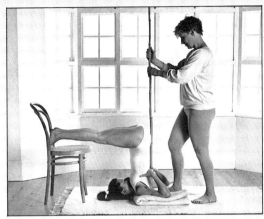

Here, too, your partner's spine should align with the pole. If her back collapses and pushes it away, she should lift her feet higher.

Basic stretch (pp. 42-3)

Reach *forwards with your arms*

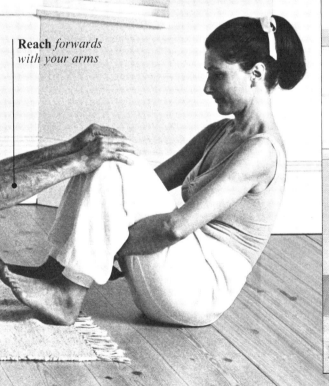

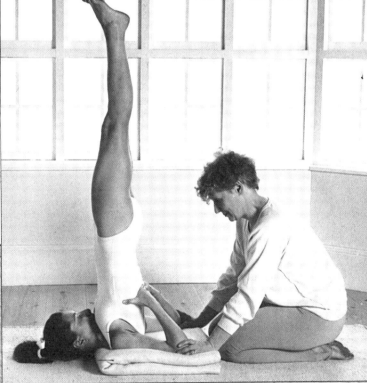

You can help your partner to get a good lift in her upper back by gently holding her elbows down and keeping them the same distance apart as her shoulders.

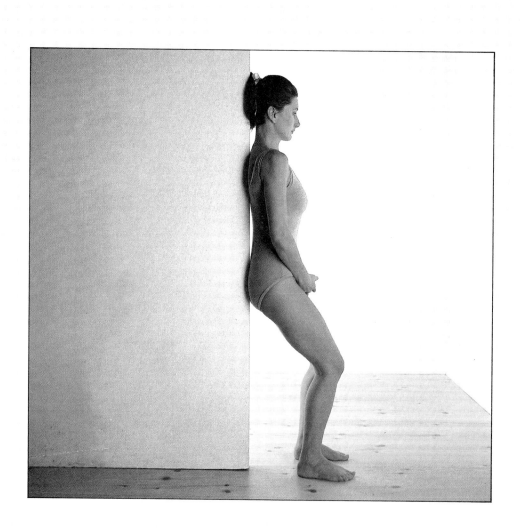

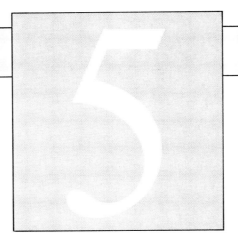

·RELIEVING·STIFFNESS·

T he perfect body is the exception, not the rule. The mere fact of being right or left handed causes uneven muscular development, so that very few people stand really well or move as easily as they might do. If you do the same actions day after day, you develop certain patterns of movement and inevitably you under-use your potential range. Your posture deteriorates and imperceptibly stiffness becomes habitual.

As long as you are healthy and carefree, you can stay blissfully unaware of the ill effects of poor posture. Most of the time you feel all right, because your body is highly adaptive and compensates with strong muscles taking over the work of weaker ones. As soon as you are tired, ill or emotionally upset, however, you become conscious of the strain. Stretching sensibly each way every day should help, but particular problems will benefit from the stretches in this chapter.

Part of the trouble stems from the way the human body has evolved. Originally designed for life on all fours, the human animal turned into a biped, and in the process major skeletal changes took place. The pelvis tilted backwards, and the new need to reach up and use hands caused the concave lumbar curve to develop. Eventually the spine developed four curves (see page 92), because a curved spine is stronger, more flexible and better able to withstand gravity than a straight one. Unfortunately, careless use of the body can upset the balance of the spinal curves. As a result, many people suffer from backache or related problems at some stage. This chapter starts with the spine, and goes on to discuss each part of the body, helping you to understand your posture and discover your areas of stiffness. Learn to use your body correctly, and enjoy the freedom that a greater range of movement brings.

The stretches in this chapter are all intended to be done before your daily stretch programme. Some are easy, others may seem a little more difficult, especially if a friend is checking you with a pole as you stretch (see Chapter Four). Go gently and use your common sense when you try the stretches. If in any doubt at all, take medical advice before you start. Remember, too, that relaxation and stretch go together. You will discover your tensions and areas of stiffness while relaxing as well as while stretching, so treat relaxation as an essential part of relieving stiffness.

·SPINE·

The spine is a wonderful piece of engineering. It manages to be both flexible and stable at the same time. Rather like a ship's mast, the spinal column is inserted into the pelvic "deck" and rises up to the head, supporting the shoulder girdle on the way, just as the mast supports the weight of the sails. Muscles and fibrous bands known as ligaments hold it in place. This structure allows the body to stabilize itself as it moves.

What causes backache?
Unfortunately, the spine's flexibility can be restricted by incorrect usage, giving rise to a number of back problems. A sudden twist at an awkward angle or an excessive strain on one part of the spine can have a painful effect on the spinal column as well as on its muscles and ligaments. To complicate things further, the core of the central nervous system, the spinal cord, runs through a channel along the length of the spine, from the top of the neck to the lumbar region. Because of this, trouble with a vertebra can put pressure on a part of the nervous system. Back problems can therefore be a cause of pain in almost any part of the body.

Most backaches have no obvious causes – but poor posture certainly contributes to back pain. If you stand well, sit straight, lie on a firm bed, wear flat shoes and lift heavy objects by bending at the knees, you are doing what you can to protect your back. The next three pages describe some common postural faults, along with good stretches to correct them. Pages 96-7 suggest a programme of stretches to ease backache, while pages 98-9 introduce some common specific back problems, with suggestions for stretches to relieve them.

·THE SPINAL COLUMN·
The spine, or backbone, stretches from the bottom of the buttocks up to the base of the skull. It is made up of more than 30 bones, known as vertebrae. The vertebrae are linked by fibrous ligaments and powerful muscles, which make the whole structure strong and flexible. The vertebrae also protect the spinal cord, which is the central channel of the nervous system.

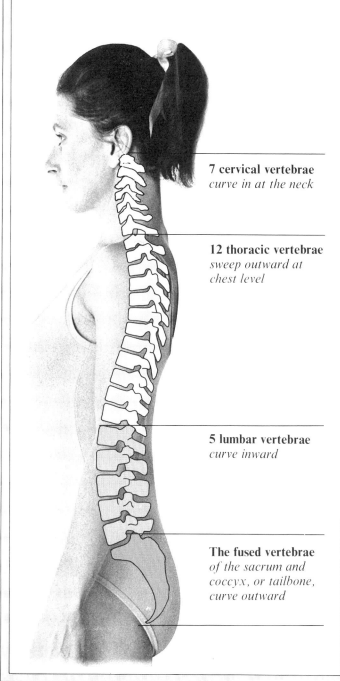

7 cervical vertebrae
curve in at the neck

12 thoracic vertebrae
sweep outward at chest level

5 lumbar vertebrae
curve inward

The fused vertebrae
of the sacrum and coccyx, or tailbone, curve outward

Good posture

Stand against a wall or door, and look in a mirror. If you are standing well, your spine will curve in at your neck and waist, out at your upper back and sacrum. There should be small gaps between your body and the door at the back of your neck and the back of your waist.

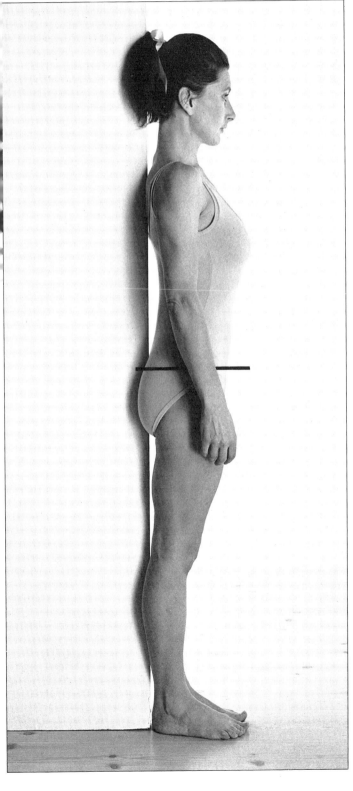

Identifying your back type

Every object has a centre of gravity with its weight evenly balanced around that centre. In the human body the centre lies inside the upper part of the pelvis, a little higher in a man than a woman. When everything is as it should be, the curves of the spine are well balanced and the pelvis is horizontal (below left). Two very common types of incorrect posture are shown below, and the black lines show that the pelvis is no longer horizontal.

Checking your posture

At first understanding comes from seeing, because a habitually faulty posture *feels* correct. Look in a mirror at your own spine from the side. Notice how you hold your shoulders and head, whether you push the back of your waist in deeply and whether your abdomen sags. Be critical of yourself. If it is difficult to see properly in a mirror, you could ask someone else to check you (see pages 76-7), or you could try standing against the edge of a door with your heels touching it. The next page shows how to correct poor posture.

Sway back

Flat back

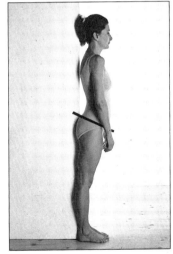 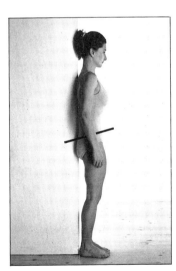

This defect is more common in women, often because high-heeled shoes pitch the body weight forwards. Because the body weight is taken by the toes, if the spinal muscles are weak the pelvis tilts forwards. The top part of the trunk then sways back, causing an excessive curve at the waist.

A flat back is more common in men. The pelvis is tilted up at the front so that there is hardly any lumbar curve. Rounded shoulders and a weak spine are part of this droopy look. It results in a rigid, more readily damaged spine, as well as causing breathing and digestive troubles.

·CORRECTING·POSTURE·

Poor posture can be corrected by strengthening back and abdominal muscles. It will take time before you feel the change in your body, but for a little effort you will be rewarded by good posture, which feels right, looks good and helps your whole body to function better.

Start by thinking tall. Lift up from your pelvis, tuck in your tailbone, extend your spine and drop your shoulders. Do the following stretches, as appropriate, every day, concentrating on feeling the changes in your muscles as you stretch. In time good posture will become second nature.

Stretch for a sway back
Rest your back against the edge of a door, with your knees bent and your feet 15-20 cm (6-9in) away from the door. There should be as little space as possible between the back of your waist and the door (right). Relax the muscles in the hollow of your waist and take a few deep breaths. Slowly straighten your knees and slide your spine up the door, tightening your abdominal muscles to keep your back flat (far right). You should feel your upper spine lift up, while your waist stays long at the back. Hold for a few seconds, then gently bend your knees and repeat two or three times.

Next you can try the stretch with your heels closer to the door, as long as you avoid increasing the gap at your waist.

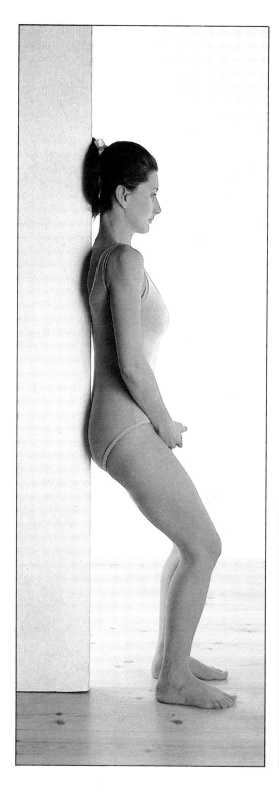
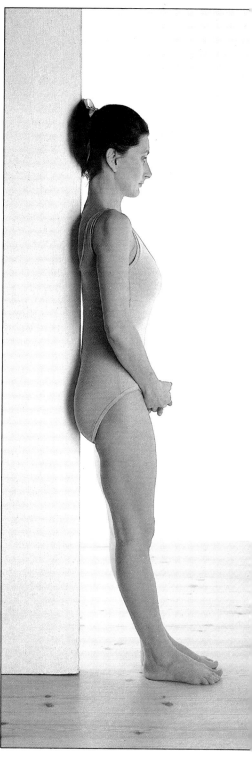

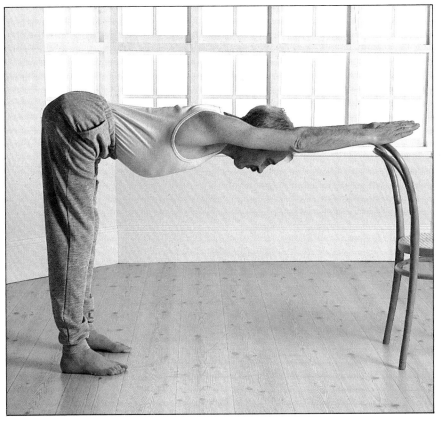

Stretch for a flat back
Tight back thigh muscles (hamstrings) often contribute to a flat back. To stretch your hamstrings, stand with your feet apart, legs straight, and bend forwards so that your hands touch the back of a chair. Lift up your bottom towards the ceiling (left). You should feel a slight dip in the back of your waist. (If your hands are too low, your waist will hump up.) Hold for a few seconds, breathing normally. Breathe in and come up. To help you lift your bottom and hollow your back, bend your knees slightly (below).

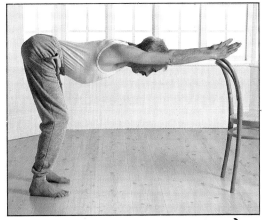

Stretch for a flat back
If you can do the upside down stretches (see pp. 42-7), you can use this position to help your waist to move in correctly. Lie on the floor with your head under the front of a chair. Then raise your back and legs so that you can rest your knees on the chair seat, using cushions if necessary for comfort. Keep your back straight. Your hips should be directly above your shoulders. Lift up your hips by pressing down on the seat with your knees, and try to pull in the back of your waist at the same time. Hold for a few minutes before bringing your legs gently down again.

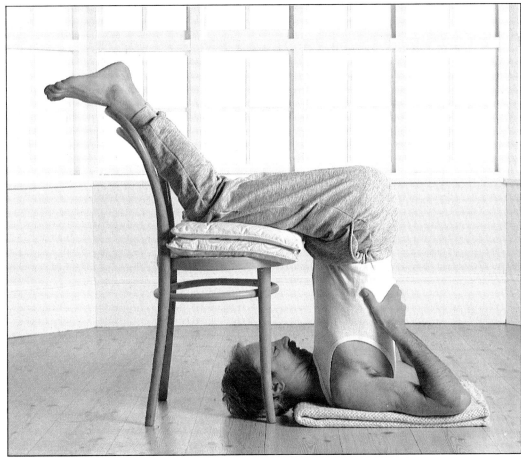

·BACKACHE·

If you have severe backache, don't start stretching without consulting your doctor. Although exercise may well form part of the treatment, you should obtain a proper diagnosis first. Specific back problems are discussed on pages 98-9.

The cause of most backaches, however, is not easily identifiable. You may have strained a muscle or ligament, there may be pressure on a nerve or you may even be suffering from stress. Daily stretching can prevent and relieve a lot of back pain. Apart from the stretches shown here, all the standing stretches from Chapter One are good for stretching and toning the muscles of the spine and abdomen. The first "less stretch twist" position is also excellent (see page 36).

If your backache is worse at the end of the day, you may need to relax before stretching. If so, lie on your back with your knees bent (see pages 50-1). This tilts your pelvis backwards and eases pressure on your lower back. Practise some deep breathing (see pages 54-5) and let the day's tensions dissolve.

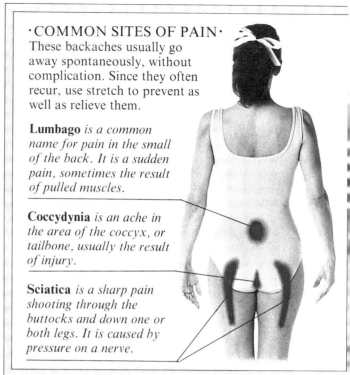

·COMMON SITES OF PAIN·
These backaches usually go away spontaneously, without complication. Since they often recur, use stretch to prevent as well as relieve them.

Lumbago *is a common name for pain in the small of the back. It is a sudden pain, sometimes the result of pulled muscles.*

Coccydynia *is an ache in the area of the coccyx, or tailbone, usually the result of injury.*

Sciatica *is a sharp pain shooting through the buttocks and down one or both legs. It is caused by pressure on a nerve.*

First stretch
This stretch eases low backache by toning the muscles of the buttocks, abdomen and thighs.

After relaxing, stay on your back with your knees bent and your arms at your sides (top right). Tighten your buttock muscles and raise your hips off the floor (bottom right). The lift should come from your hips, not your waist, and your pelvis should be higher than your navel. Hold for as long as you can, breathing normally, then breathe out and lower your hips gently to the floor.

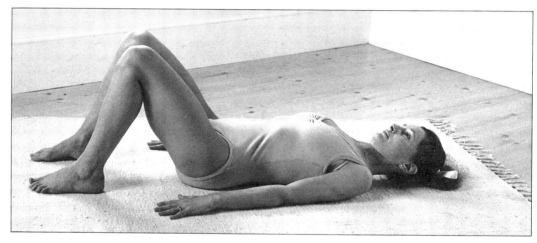

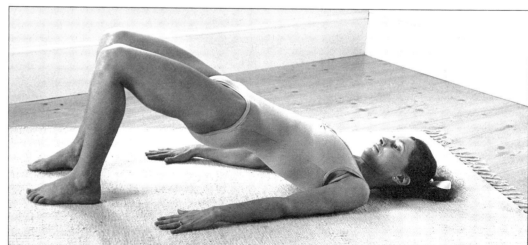

Second stretch
All you need for this stretch are a few books. Lie on the floor, knees bent, keeping your back flat and your tailbone tucked in. Tighten the muscles underneath your buttocks. Then stretch your arms above your head to lengthen your upper back, holding the books to weigh your hands down (top right). Stretch as hard as you can without arching your back. You should feel your abdominal muscles firm and flatten. Still stretching, straighten your legs (bottom right). Hold for as long as you can, breathing normally.

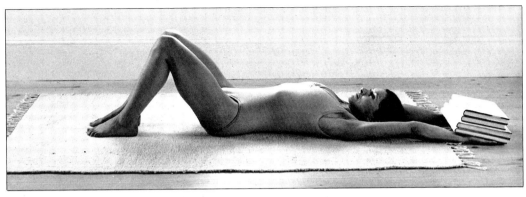

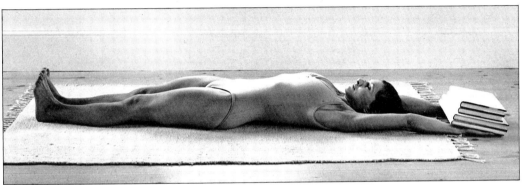

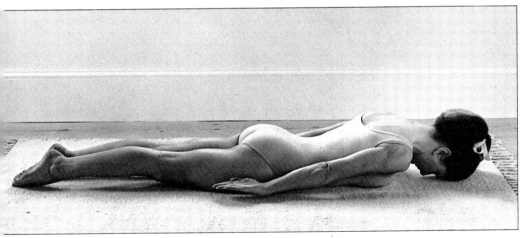

Third stretch
This stretch eases very low backache. Lie on the floor face down, with your arms at your sides, palms up (top left). Follow the instructions on p. 40, remembering not to take your head higher than your feet (bottom left). You should feel the stretch in the sacral region. Hold for a few seconds, breathe out and come down.

To make the stretch more intense, do it with your knees bent and your shins perpendicular to the floor. Start with your thighs apart and try to bring your knees together. (This is not shown.)

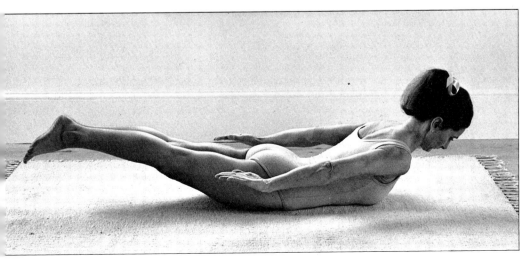

·BACK·PROBLEMS·

Three common back problems are shown here, along with some suggestions for stretches that you may find particularly helpful. These stretches should be done in the context of extending and stretching as a whole. This is because a deviation or injury in one particular part of the back affects the entire structure of your body. So when stretching to relieve a specific problem you should continue to stretch your entire spine. However, if you have a specific back problem you must take medical advice.

Scoliosis

Scoliosis is a sideways curvature of the spine. The pelvis tilts to one side and a sideways bend of the spine occurs in the pelvic area, with a compensating curve developing on the opposite side of the upper back, creating an S-shape. When the problem is severe, it is hard to remedy, and orthopaedic treatment may be necessary. If you suffer from severe scoliosis, take medical advice before you start to stretch.

Many people suffer from scoliosis to a lesser degree. If your muscles are stronger on one side, depending on whether you are right or left handed, you may well develop a slight postural imbalance. This can be corrected by stretching both sides of your body evenly. Concentrate on the "less stretch" movements, so that you can extend your spine and stretch the underdeveloped muscles on the weak side of your body. It is ideal if someone can use a pole to check your alignment (see Chapter Four).

Scoliotic posture

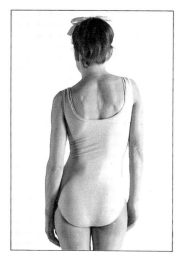

Correcting scoliosis (right)
It is particularly important to stretch correctly in the twists. Ask a friend to hold a pole vertically behind you in one of the "less stretch" positions to make sure that you turn without aggravating the scoliosis (see pp. 86-7).

·PROLAPSED DISC·
Flexible discs made of cartilage lie between the vertebrae to cushion the bone and allow spinal movement. Discs are not supplied with nerves or blood. But they can cause acute pain if they prolapse (perhaps because you are overstraining your spine). A prolapsed disc (right), more commonly known as a slipped disc, requires medical attention. However, standing straight and stretching correctly in most positions is still beneficial.
Caution: You should avoid all forwards stretches if your condition is acute, because bending forwards can increase pressure on the affected nerve. For the same reason, do not do the basic upside down stretch; do the "less stretch upside down" movement instead.

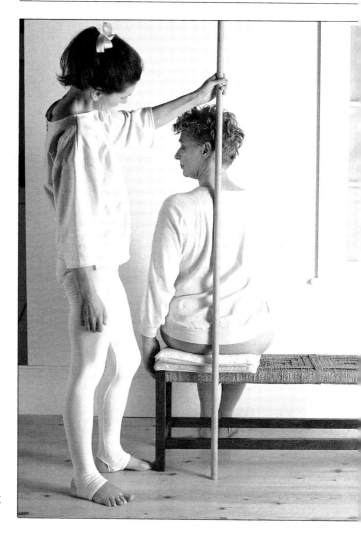

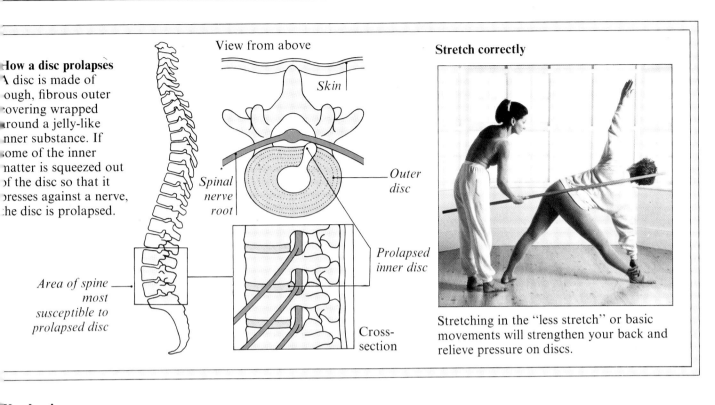

How a disc prolapses
A disc is made of tough, fibrous outer covering wrapped around a jelly-like inner substance. If some of the inner matter is squeezed out of the disc so that it presses against a nerve, the disc is prolapsed.

View from above

Skin

Spinal nerve root

Outer disc

Prolapsed inner disc

Cross-section

Area of spine most susceptible to prolapsed disc

Stretch correctly

Stretching in the "less stretch" or basic movements will strengthen your back and relieve pressure on discs.

Kyphosis

Kyphosis is an outward curve of the upper spine that causes hunched, rounded shoulders. It is often the result of degenerating vertebrae, muscles and ligaments in old age.

If you have kyphosis, the outward curve of your upper back will make your neck curve in and your head drop forward. When you stretch, try to extend the back of your neck so that the back of your skull comes into line. All the stretches in Chapter One are beneficial, especially the twists (see pages 34-7). When relaxing, you should put a cushion under your head (see page 52).

Correcting kyphosis
Lie on the floor with a folded blanket or rug under your shoulders and elbows. With your knees bent and your feet on the seat of a chair, hold the front legs of the chair (below left). Take a few deep breaths. On an out-breath, press your feet down on the front of the chair seat and lift up your hips (below right). Stretch up your spine, extending your neck and tucking in your chin. Use your feet to lift up your hips so that your upper back extends and straightens. Hold for a few seconds, breathing normally. Breathe out, come down and repeat once or twice.

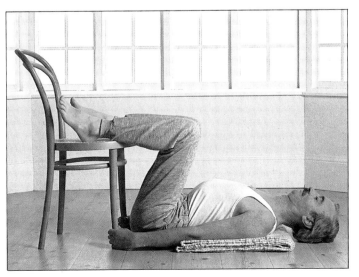

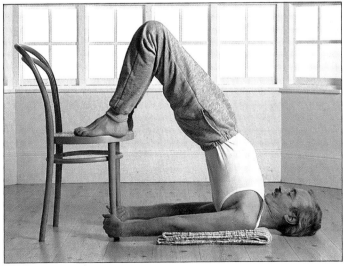

· UPPER · BODY ·

Consisting of the head, the neck, the shoulders, the upper back, the arms and the hands, the upper body is an extremely mobile structure, vulnerable to distortion by muscular tension.

If the weight of the head is carried correctly on top of the spine, the neck can move freely. However, very often the head is carried slightly off balance. The muscles on one side of the neck tighten; as a result tightness round the neck and shoulders can cause breathing problems, as well as affecting movement of arms and hands.

When you stand properly, with your shoulders free and your chest open, your arms and hands relax and you use your fingers and wrists with ease. When you are stiff across the shoulders and neck, your hands and wrists also feel tight and tense. To ease stiffness, look at the stretches on the next five pages.

·STRUCTURE OF THE UPPER BODY·

The whole bony upper body is lighter and more mobile than the weight-supporting hips, legs and lower spine. The vertebrae become smaller at the top of the spine, allowing the neck to turn easily. The shoulder girdle is attached by ligaments only to the thorax, where the collar bones meet the top of the breast bone, allowing it to glide freely over the ribcage. The ribcage is very elastic, as the curving ribs, which hang from the spine at the back, attach to the breast bone through cartilage. This enables the ribcage to expand and contract with the breath.

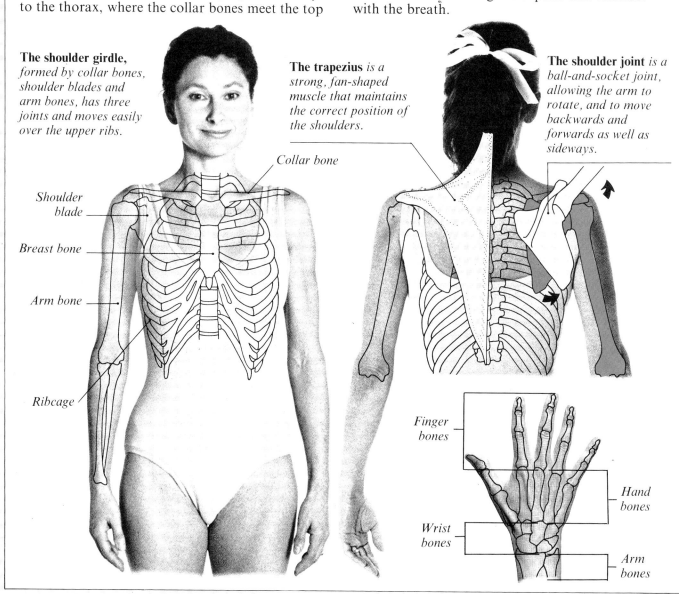

The shoulder girdle, *formed by collar bones, shoulder blades and arm bones, has three joints and moves easily over the upper ribs.*

The trapezius *is a strong, fan-shaped muscle that maintains the correct position of the shoulders.*

The shoulder joint *is a ball-and-socket joint, allowing the arm to rotate, and to move backwards and forwards as well as sideways.*

Collar bone

Shoulder blade

Breast bone

Arm bone

Ribcage

Finger bones

Hand bones

Wrist bones

Arm bones

· HEAD & NECK ·

The way you habitually hold your head affects the amount of wear and tear on the small vertebrae and discs in your neck. Very often the neck muscles tighten. Tension in the neck is a common cause of headache.

If your neck is stiff, you will find the sideways stretches and the twists difficult. Relieve tension by doing one or more of the movements on this page before you do your usual stretch programme. Make sure you use a thick folded blanket under your shoulders in the upside down stretches. When relaxing, use a small cushion under your head.

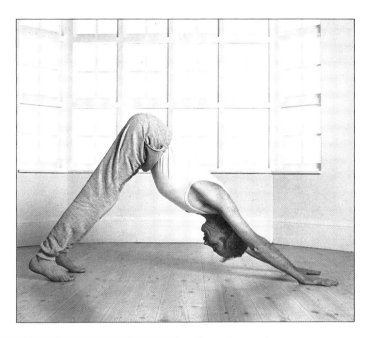

First stretch
Kneel on all fours. Lifting your bottom up and extending your spine, straighten your arms and legs. Let your chest open and your shoulders release. Let your head hang freely. Keep your throat and face relaxed. Hold for at least a minute before returning to all fours.

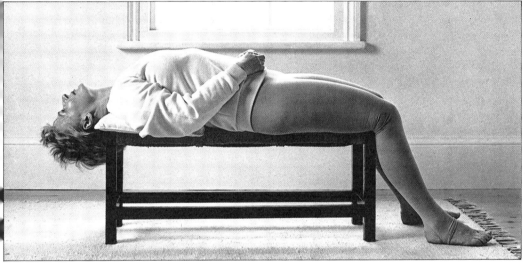

Second stretch
This stretch can be done lying on a bed or low table. Lie so that the back of your head is just off the edge of the table, using a cushion to extend the curve of your neck. You should feel a gentle stretch in your neck, but no tension in your eyes or forehead. Hold for a minute and support your head with your hands as you come up.

Third stretch
This "more stretch forwards" movement is an excellent one in which to let the weight of your head help stretch your neck (see p. 33). Either hold your elbows (far right) or let your arms hang down heavily from the shoulders (right). Hold for a minute, breathe in and come up.

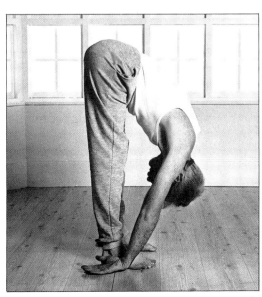

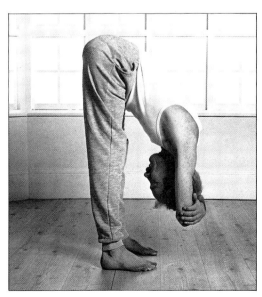

·SHOULDERS·

The shoulder joints are the most mobile joints in your body. Consisting of collar bones at the front, arm bones, and shoulder blades at the back, your shoulder joints allow your arms to move in almost any direction (see page 100). Problems frequently arise because over a period of time this range of movement becomes restricted.

A rounded back and stiff shoulders are often the result of poor posture over many years. Most occupations require a lot of forward bending, as people stoop over desks, workbenches, babies, drawing boards or kitchen sinks. The tendency when bending forwards with the neck unsupported is to tighten the trapezius muscle (the strong fan-shaped muscle behind the top of the shoulders and neck – see page 100). You may find yourself doing this without noticing it, to stop yourself tilting forwards. After a time this tightening of the neck and shoulders becomes a habit, and the muscle fails to release completely even when you are no longer bending forwards. Eventually your whole upper trunk and neck may become distorted.

In many older people there is an increase in the curve of the upper back, causing the shoulders to push forwards and the chest to cave in. Tension in the shoulders then hinders the movement of the ribs and affects breathing (see page 55).

Once established, the habit of tightening your shoulders is extremely difficult to correct, as it becomes second nature to round your shoulders every time you stand or sit. The stretches on these pages have been designed to loosen stiffness in the muscles slowly, gradually restoring a full range of movement. Ideally you should do the whole range of stretches every day immediately before your regular practice session (see pages 58-73). Practise the movements slowly and carefully, aiming to increase your range little by little. The shoulders should never be forced or wrenched. If you have ever injured or dislocated your shoulders, consult your doctor before doing the stretches.

The stretches on the next two pages can all be done standing, or in a sitting position. At first you may feel your muscles tense and tighten as you stretch. Hold each position for a second or two only and then repeat it. As your shoulders become looser you will find that you can gradually build up the time you hold each stretch. Start the sequence by relaxing your shoulders as much as you can (below). The stretches will come more easily if you take a little time over this first.

Relaxing your shoulders
Kneel on a folded blanket or rug. Let your head rest comfortably on some cushions or pillows in front of you, perhaps raised on a low stool. Fold your arms and hold your elbows, leaning forwards so that your elbows are slightly higher than your head. As you relax forwards you will feel a gentle stretch in your shoulders. Do *not* try to press down in this position; simply relax and on every out-breath feel the tension in your shoulders gradually easing.

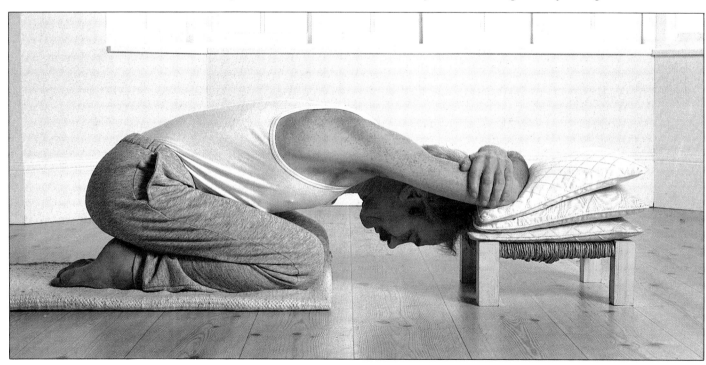

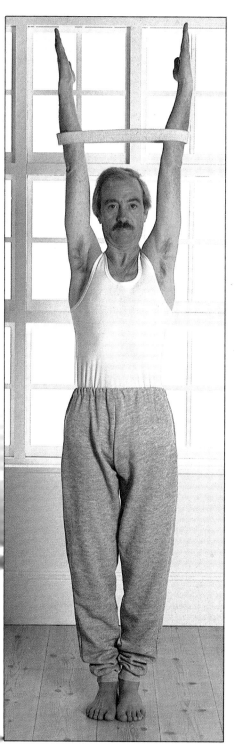

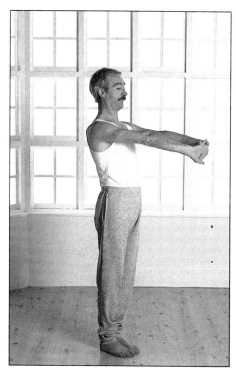

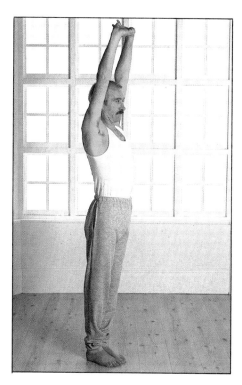

Second stretch
Link your fingers and turn your palms out. Bring your arms up to shoulder level, elbows straight. On a deep out-breath stretch your arms up above your head. Stretch your wrists and open your palms. Repeat with opposite thumb on top.

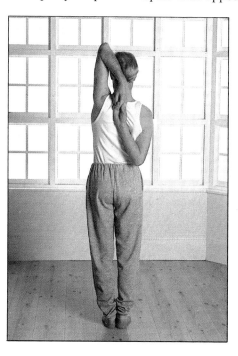

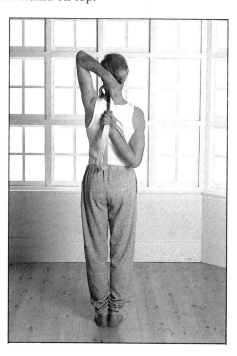

First stretch
Tie a belt around your elbows so that when you push against it your elbows are as wide apart as your shoulders. Take your arms above your head, palms facing each other, and keep your elbows straight. Push outwards against the belt. You will feel the stretch in your shoulders.

Third stretch
Bend your right elbow so your hand rests vertically on your spine, palm out. Breathing in stretch your left arm over your head; breathing out bend your elbow and catch your hands or, if this is hard, a belt. Repeat, hands the other way round.

·SHOULDERS·

Stretching forwards

If you are doing a beginners' or basic programme, do these two shoulder stretches sitting as shown. If you usually do a "more stretch" programme, you could try stretching forwards standing, keeping your legs straight.

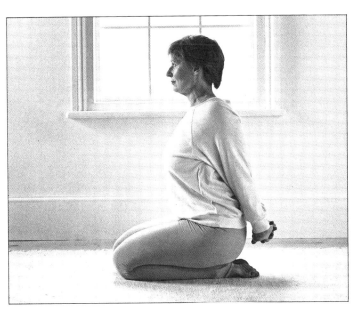

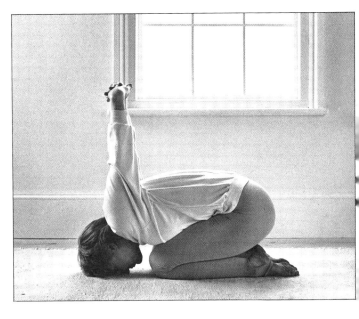

Fourth stretch

1 Kneel and sit on your heels, then clasp your hands together behind your back. (If you find this hard at first, hold a belt instead.) Open your chest and straighten your elbows. Take a few breaths, then breathe in deeply.

2 On an out-breath, bend forwards. Keeping your bottom on your heels, stretch your arms back and up as you go down. Rest your chest on your thighs. (If your knees are stiff, put a cushion on your heels under your hips.)

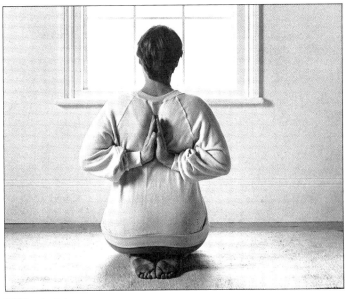

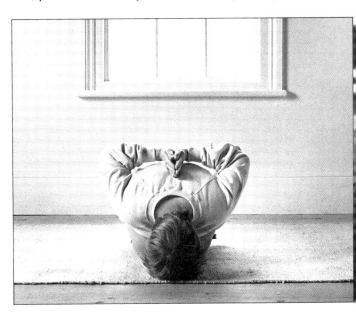

Fifth stretch

1 Kneel and sit on your heels. Take your hands behind your back, palms together and fingers pointing down. Then point your fingers up, still with palms together, and try to take your elbows back. Hold for a few seconds.

2 Take a deep breath in and bend forwards as you breathe out. Keep your elbows back so that all your fingers and your thumbs touch as you go down. Hold for a few seconds, breathing normally, then breathe in and come up.

· HANDS ·

Your fingers are normally slightly curled when relaxed, and they tend to stiffen in this position. The stretches on this page will loosen stiff fingers, hands and wrists. Do them daily for a few months and your hands will become more flexible.

First stretch
If your fingers are stiff and hard to straighten, they need a little help. Gently extend them back one by one (right). Then take them all back at the same time (far right). This helps to stretch open your palm. Repeat several times.

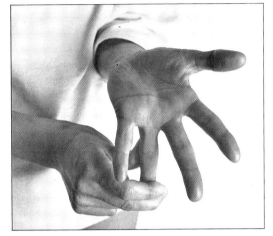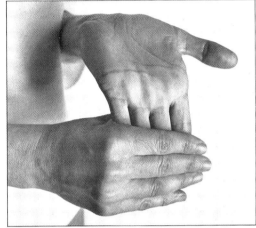

Second stretch
Take your thumb back towards your wrist (right). Then bring it forwards, stretching gently and firmly (far right). Never force it. Finish by making a fist and slowly opening it, stretching your fingers and thumb out as far as you can.

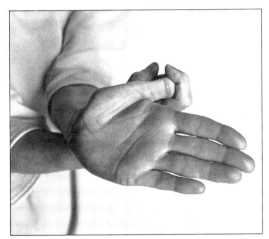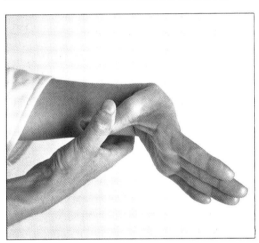

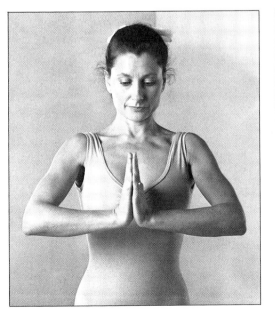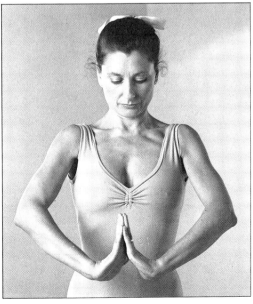

Third stretch
Put your palms together, fingers pointing upwards, as if you were praying. Stretch your fingers and press palms together strongly. Keep the base of your palms pressing together, as you gradually lower your hands until your lower arms are horizontal (far left). Then take your hands down still further, fingers and upper palms together (left). You should feel the stretch on the insides of your fingers and wrists. Hold for a few seconds, then repeat.

· HIPS ·

If you have flexible hip joints, you should have no difficulty in moving your legs backwards and forwards, swinging them away from and across your body and rotating them in and out. Without your feeling any strain on your spine, your pelvis can adjust easily and support the weight of your upper body as you walk, stand and run.

Unfortunately, freedom of movement in the hip joints is a casualty of western civilization. People living without furniture, without fitted kitchens or bathrooms, spend a lot of time squatting and sitting on the floor. Their flexibility and ease of movement are in striking contrast with the stiffness of adults in the west. Your child may squat happily to play but, if you spend your days sitting in chairs or cars, you very quickly lose the ability to rotate your thighs.

During the first half of your life this may not seem to matter. But hips that are not fully used develop tight muscles. In time, uneven pressure on the joints causes wear and tear, commonly known as arthritis or osteoarthritis. This in turn leads to further restricted movement. Stiffness and pain in the joints mean that you use them even less, and slowly the muscles begin to waste away. It is a vicious circle: use your hip joints properly when you can, or there may come a time when you can't.

Many sports – including jogging, ski-ing and cycling – involve restricted hip movement. Stretch, on the other hand, actively promotes flexible hips. All the basic stretches from Chapter One will ease stiffness in the muscles surrounding the hip joints. (You should pay particular attention to the position of your feet on the floor in the standing stretches and, where your legs are straight, keep your knees strongly extended to ensure you feel the stretch correctly.) All the stretches on these three pages are designed to improve the rotation of the thighs. Stretch will help you – either to maintain flexible hips or to loosen stiff ones.

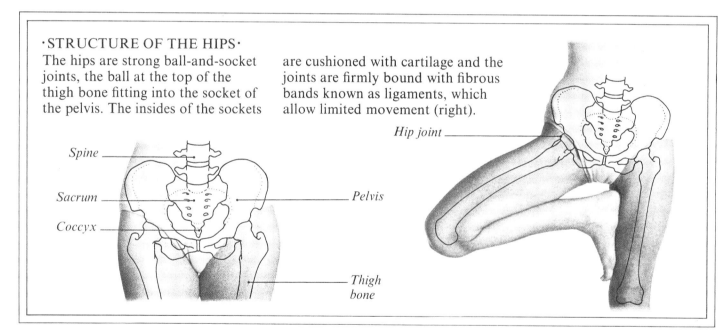

·STRUCTURE OF THE HIPS·
The hips are strong ball-and-socket joints, the ball at the top of the thigh bone fitting into the socket of the pelvis. The insides of the sockets are cushioned with cartilage and the joints are firmly bound with fibrous bands known as ligaments, which allow limited movement (right).

Hip joint

Spine

Sacrum

Coccyx

Pelvis

Thigh bone

First stretch
To test the flexibility of your hips and to give them a good stretch, lie on your back and bend your knees. Taking your feet towards your buttocks, soles together, let your knees fall outwards. Your weight should be evenly distributed so that both knees are the same distance from the floor.

If your knees do not easily fall outwards, try this stretch with your feet raised on cushions (right). Have the soles of your feet against each other and relax into the stretch for a few minutes every day.

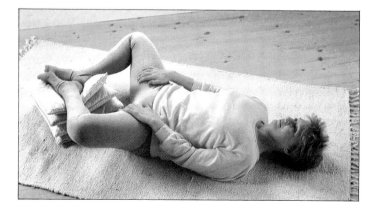

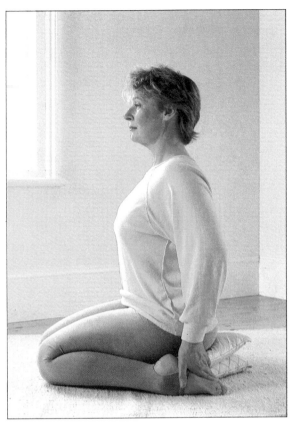

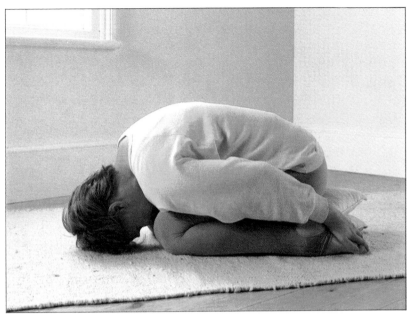

Second stretch
Sit on cushions between your feet, keeping your knees together (left). If this feels easy, try bending forwards, keeping your bottom on the cushions (above). As the position becomes more comfortable, you can remove a cushion at a time, until after a few weeks you are sitting on the floor.

Third stretch
Sit on the floor and cross one knee over the other. With your hands on the floor for support, sit as tall as you can. Hold for a few seconds, then repeat with your knees the other way round.

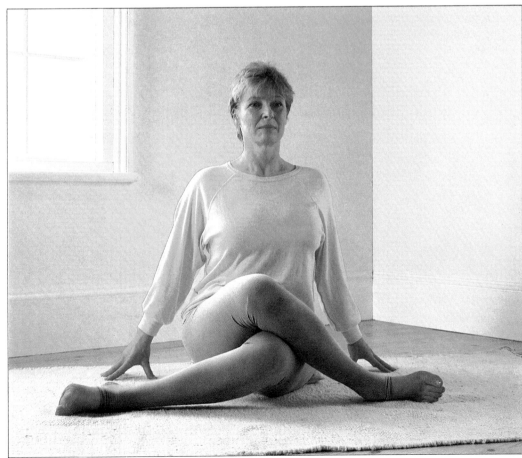

· HIPS ·

Stretching upside down
In the upside down positions, the hip joints do not have to support the weight of your body while you are stretching and working them. This is especially useful if you suffer from arthritis in your hips.

Before you attempt the stretches on this page, however, you must be able to maintain the basic upside down position comfortably and securely for some minutes (see pages 42-3). If possible, ask someone to help position the chair and books.

Fourth stretch

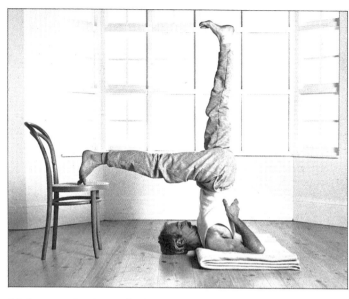

Fifth stretch

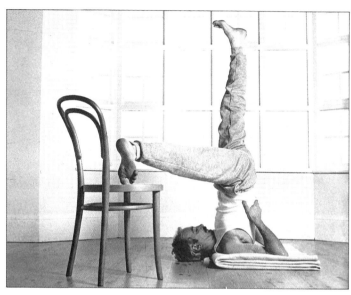

Make your body vertical, resting your neck and shoulders on a folded rug or blanket. Extend your body in the basic inverted position. As you stretch, lower one leg and rest your foot on a chair behind your head. Your back and hips should stay straight. Hold for up to 30 seconds, keeping both knees straight. Then stretch both legs up again, and repeat with the other leg. When you find this easy, try taking your foot down a little more, on to a stool or a pile of books.

When you have mastered the previous stretch, try taking your leg out to the side. Again start with a straight back and both legs stretching up. Turn one leg out as far as possible before you start taking it out to the side and lowering it on to a chair. How far sideways you can take your leg will depend on the outward rotation of your thighs. Make sure you have the chair in the right place. Keep your knees straight and your body vertical. Hold for up to 30 seconds, then stretch up and repeat with the other leg.

Sixth stretch
Again start with a straight back and both legs stretching up. Keeping your knees straight, slowly take both legs out to the side and lower them on to a low table or on to two piles of books. Lift your hips and stretch the backs of your legs. Hold for up to 30 seconds and bend your knees to come up.

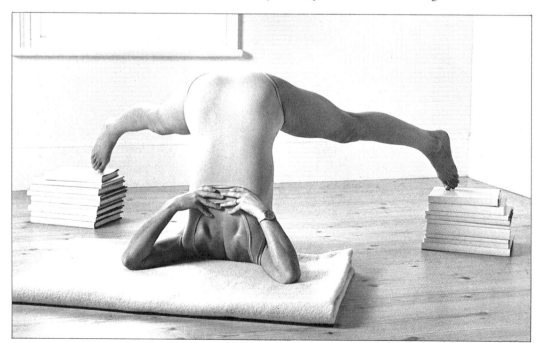

· KNEES & LEGS ·

Knees are the most vulnerable parts of legs, and accidents and injuries are the cause of most knee problems. The construction of the knee is complicated: criss-crossing ligaments hold the joint in place, while pads of cartilage act as shock absorbers between the bones. If wear and tear on the knee joint is uneven and the muscles weaken, a sudden blow or awkward movement can cause the cartilage to tear and slip out of place. It is also possible to stand so that the backs of your legs become overstretched (right).

Stretching is perfect exercise for knees and legs, although you should first take medical advice if you have ever injured your knees. If your leg muscles are aching and tired by the end of the day, or if you have varicose veins, the upside down stretches in particular are a wonderful antidote (see pages 42-7). The stretches on the next two pages are designed to strengthen the muscles around the knees, especially the front thigh muscles.

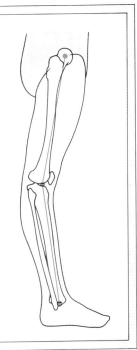

·OVERSTRETCHED LEG·

When you stand with your legs straight, your weight should fall on the centre of your hip joints, knees and ankles (below). If you are overstretching your legs as you stand, the extra strain on the backs of your knees weakens the ligaments behind them (right).

To correct overstretched legs, keep your weight more over the balls of your feet instead of on your heels, and never push into the back of your knees when you are stretching. Lift your front thigh muscles instead.

·STRUCTURE OF THE LEG·

The leg consists of four bones. The femur, or thigh bone, connects the hip to the knee, and is the longest and strongest bone in the body. At its lower end it forms part of the knee joint. A small, flat, triangular bone, the patella, or kneecap, makes a hinge at the front that protects the knee joint. Below the knee are two leg bones. The tibia, or shin bone, runs from the front of the knee to the ankle, forming part of both the knee and the ankle joints. The fibula lies on the outer side of the tibia and forms part of the ankle joint at its lower end.

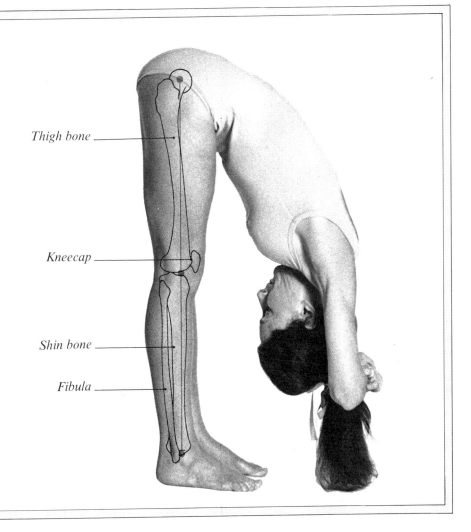

Thigh bone

Kneecap

Shin bone

Fibula

·KNEES & LEGS·

Even if the knee joint has been weakened, it can still be partly protected by strengthening the muscles around it. The three stretches on these pages improve the muscle tone of the thighs.

First stretch

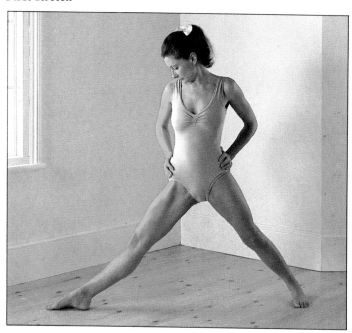

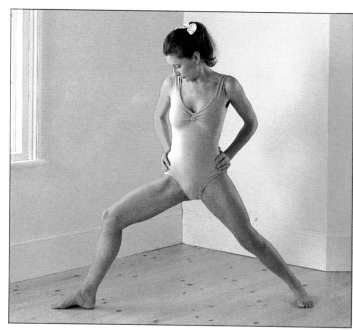

1 With your hands on your hips, take your feet wide apart. Turn your left foot slightly in and your right leg out. The centre of your right knee should face out to the right, in line with your right foot. Spread out your toes, lifting the arch of your right foot. Pull up your right kneecap by tightening your front thigh muscles.

2 Resisting with your shin, bend your right knee a little. Continue to keep your knee in line with your foot. Hold for a few seconds, pulling up your kneecap. Relax your muscles and bend your knee a little more, still resisting with your shin. Hold for a few more seconds, again pulling up your front thigh muscles.

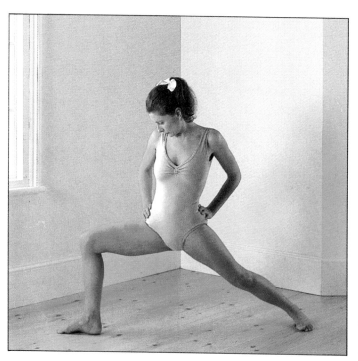

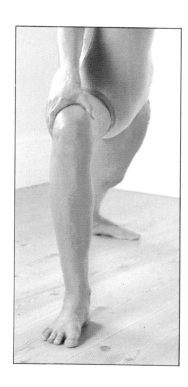

3 Continue to bend your right knee little by little, until your right thigh is parallel to the floor and your shin is at a right angle to it (left). At each stage, make sure that the centre of your knee is still in line with the centre of your foot (right). Come up slowly and repeat on the other side.

Second stretch

Stand with your back against a wall, your feet slightly in front of you and about 15 cm (6 in) apart. Your legs should be straight and your feet parallel to each other, pointing forwards. Bend your knees slightly without turning them out. Keeping your back straight, slide down the wall a little. Hold for a count of five. With your feet still pointing forwards, bend your knees a little more and again hold for a count of five. Keeping your heels down on the floor and your arches lifted, go down in stages as far as you can. Then come up slowly in the same way, holding for a count of five at each pause.

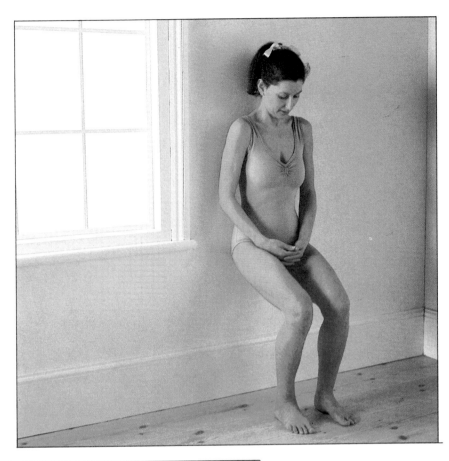

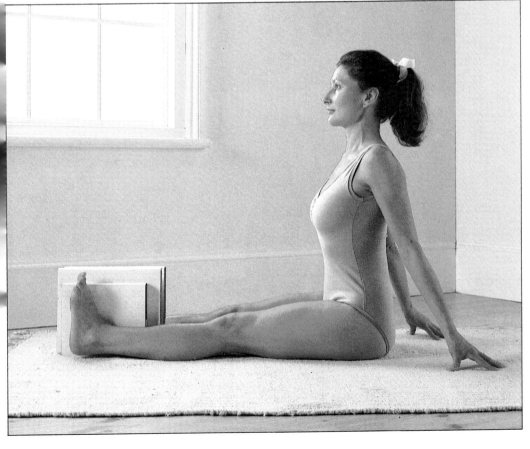

Third stretch

Sit on a rug on the floor, with your back and legs straight, and your hands behind your back touching the floor for extra support. (Sit on a cushion if your lower back sags.) Stretch out your legs, extending your heels. If your ankles touch while your knees are far apart, put a book between your ankles and stretch the insides of your heels and your big toes to help them straighten. Then tighten your front thigh muscles and pull up your kneecaps. Both your knees should be working strongly: if one side is weaker than the other, work it a little harder. Hold for a few seconds, then relax. Repeat several times.

·FEET & ANKLES·

Feet should be strong and flexible, with the toes evenly spaced so that as you walk they spread out on the floor for balance. Although your feet are a very small base of support for your body, they are well designed to do the job of bearing your weight. However, it is most important that you stand well, because faults allowed to develop in the feet have postural repercussions throughout the body.

Stand on a dry, smooth surface with wet feet and see what impression you make. Your toes, heels and soles should press the floor and leave a print. If the print of one foot is better than the other, your weight is not evenly distributed and you should give a little time to standing straight (see page 17). If your arches leave a print, you are suffering from fallen arches. Although flat feet are common in early childhood, in later life fallen arches are frequently the cause of tired, aching feet. This is because your arches hold the bones of your feet and ankles in their correct positions and encourage your foot muscles to function normally. They also act as shock absorbers. If they have fallen, your muscles and ligaments endure extra stress.

Otherwise, problems with feet are mostly caused by shoes. Fashion in shoes takes little account of the needs of feet. Even low heels throw body weight forwards on to the balls of the feet, making the backs of your ankles tight and stiff. Ill-fitting shoes push toes together and often cause corns and calluses to develop. In extreme cases shoes even make toes cross over and sometimes this can inflame the big toe, giving rise to a painful bunion. Women are more prone than men to almost all foot problems. High heels can throw the body out of line and put excessive pressure on the balls of the feet and the toes (as well as putting the spine under great stress).

By stretching your feet, you can help to correct the damage done by poor footwear. The stretches opposite are all strengthening.

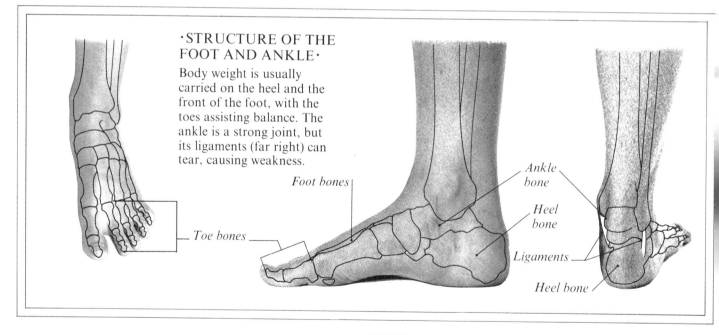

·STRUCTURE OF THE FOOT AND ANKLE·
Body weight is usually carried on the heel and the front of the foot, with the toes assisting balance. The ankle is a strong joint, but its ligaments (far right) can tear, causing weakness.

Foot bones

Toe bones

Ankle bone

Heel bone

Ligaments

Heel bone

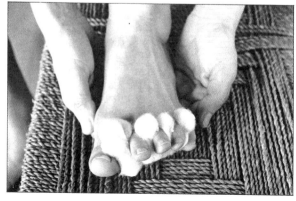

Caring for your feet
If ill-fitting shoes are deforming your toes, don't wear them. Pull your toes apart with your fingers to stretch them and put pads of cotton wool between your toes to keep them separate if necessary (right). Walk with bare feet whenever you can and always stretch barefoot.

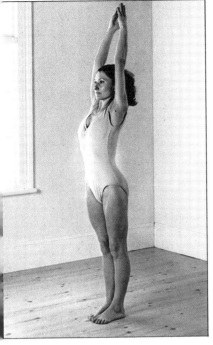
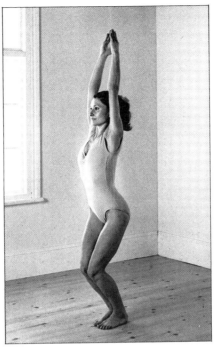

First stretch

This strengthens the muscles of the legs and ankles. Stand up straight, keeping your feet parallel and together. Stretch your arms up above your head, palms together (far left). Take a few breaths. On an out-breath, bend your knees as much as you can, without lifting your heels off the floor or bending forwards (left). Breathe in and come up. Repeat two or three times.

Second stretch

Kneel up with your feet and ankles together (right). Then sit on your heels (far right). If this is difficult, tie a belt around your ankles to keep them from separating. Stretch up through your spine, keeping your weight evenly distributed between your heels. Hold for a few minutes. If fallen arches make your feet ache, do this every day.

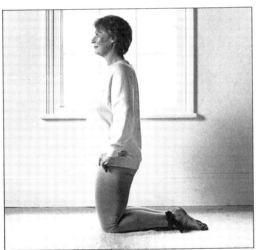
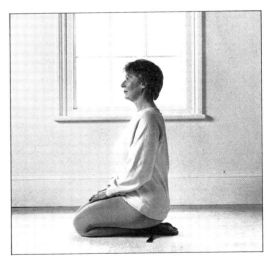

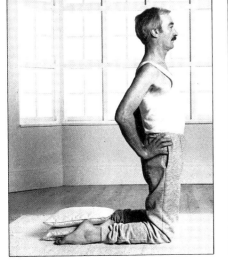
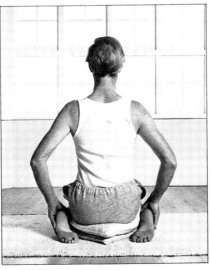

Third stretch

This also benefits your arches, as well as strengthening your ankles. Kneel up, knees together and cushions between your feet (far left). Sit on the cushions and stretch up through your spine. Then stretch the outsides of your feet towards the floor (left). Hook your thumbs inside your ankles and turn out your calves, encouraging your little toes to stretch towards the floor. Hold for a few seconds and repeat as necessary.

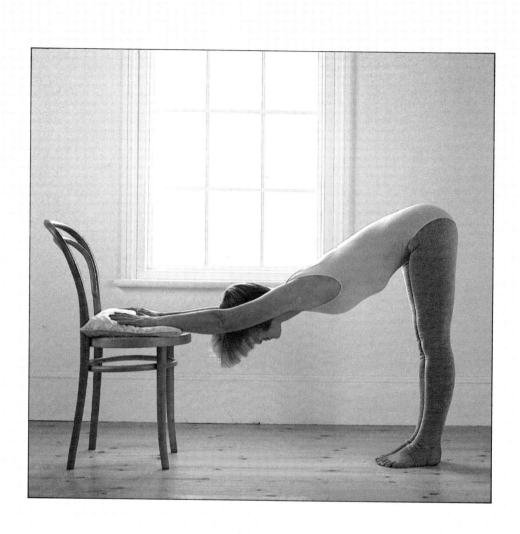

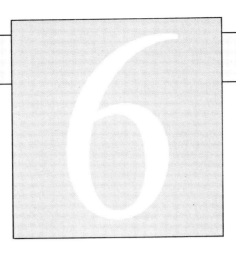

·RELIEVING·STRESS·

Because stress and stress-related problems receive a good deal of publicity, it is easy to forget that a certain amount of stress is necessary. Stress triggers the energy to create and achieve as well as to survive, a response originating with primitive man who, when alerted to danger, tensed his muscles and quickened his heart rate, preparing for flight or defence.

Nowadays it is rarely immediate physical danger that causes fear or anxiety. More often the train is late, there is pressure at work or personal relationships are proving difficult. In these circumstances you may feel the effects of stress, but not the release through physical action that your body expects to follow the tension. As frustration builds up, each crisis makes an overstressed person more vulnerable.

Life does not run smoothly all the time. Now and again everyone needs help with physical, mental or emotional stress, and there are many forms of stress relief on offer. Clever marketing convinces of the need for external remedies – whether in the form of pills, alcohol or therapy. In fact many of life's crises can be surmounted without resorting to external remedies. Helping yourself from your own resources makes you stronger and better able to cope the next time. Reaching for unnecessary stimulants and tranquillizers is weakening and breeds dependence.

With a little time and patience you can alleviate stress, in all its different forms. You may be powerless to solve the problems, but you can do a great deal to prevent them from overwhelming you. It may take surprisingly little to brighten your outlook.

For a start you can reverse the syndrome of physical tensions caused by emotional setbacks or hostile circumstances. The programmes in this chapter are designed to help you respond constructively to various types of crisis and tension.

Ideally you should be familiar with the stretches in the first chapter before you do any of these programmes, because detailed instructions for stretches described in Chapter One are not repeated here. Pay careful attention to the information in the programmes, since relieving stress by exercise is more subtle than ordinary everyday stretching.

NOTE: If a picture in this chapter shows a more advanced stretch from Chapter One than the one you would normally do, replace it by the appropriate movement at your usual stretch level. The benefits will be the same.

·STOP·CRYING·

Everybody cries sometimes. Occasional tears are no bad thing, but there always comes a time when you have to dry your eyes and get on with life. Often this is not easy, for you find yourself sobbing and gulping long after you want to stop. By doing some strong outward stretches you can prevent yourself from being overwhelmed by your emotions again as you calm down. The following positions will help you feel able to face the world.

1 Relax

Lie on your back, your body raised off the floor, perhaps on a low table, while your head and the tops of your shoulders are supported on the floor by cushions. Breathe slowly and deeply. It is essential to keep your eyes open, fixing your gaze on a point above you. Stay like this for 5 to 10 minutes. To come out of the position bend your knees and rest for a few seconds. Then slide your back gently off the stool.

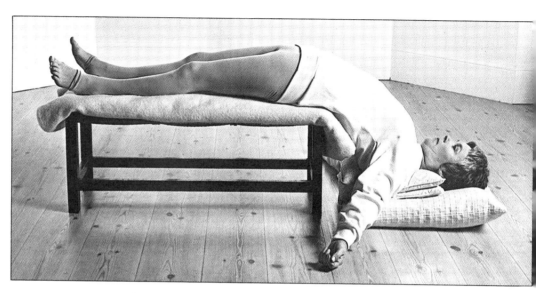

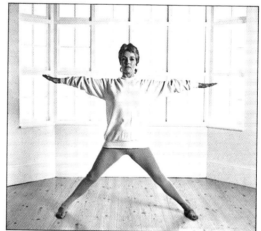

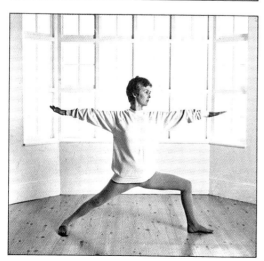

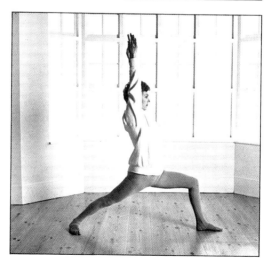

2 Wide and strong

When you feel calm enough to do some active stretching, stand up and do as many of the stretches from pp. 22-5 as you can (omitting only the second stretch on p. 25, as balancing on one leg is not helpful here). Hold each position for a few seconds, changing sides when appropriate and stretching outwards strongly. Concentrate on breathing smoothly and steadily, opening your chest as you breathe in deeply. Repeat several times. Your shoulders should feel loose and relaxed before you attempt the next positions.

3 Upside down

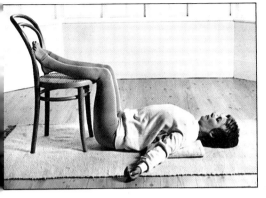

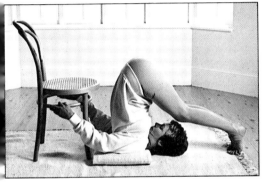

Lie on a rug on the floor, a folded blanket under your shoulders and upper arms. Rest your legs on a chair (top). Hold the chair and pull it towards you as, on an out-breath, you swing your legs over your head, lifting your upper back as much as possible (above). Take your feet down as far as you comfortably can. Pull the chair further towards you until you can hold its back legs. The seat of the chair should support your lower back when you bring your legs above your head as described on pp. 42-3 (right). Hold for up to 5 minutes before coming down slowly.

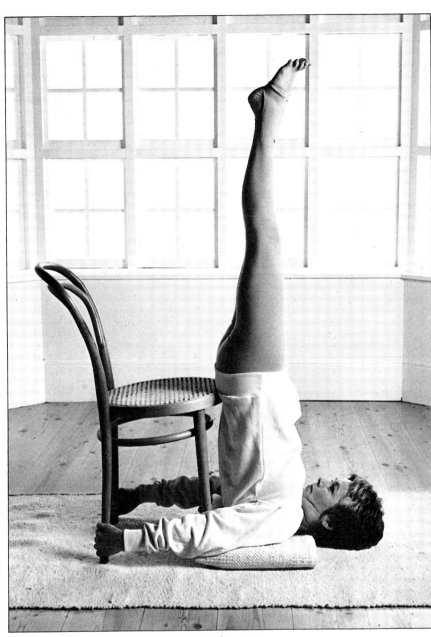

4 Relax

After finishing these active stretches, it is essential to keep your outlook positive. For this reason, do not end by relaxing with your eyes closed. If you want to rest, repeat the first position with your body raised off the floor, keeping your chest and eyes open. Breathe slowly and deeply, making your in-breath long and steady. Stay in the position for 5 to 10 minutes before bending your knees, resting for a few seconds with your feet close to your hips and sliding your back gently down off the stool.

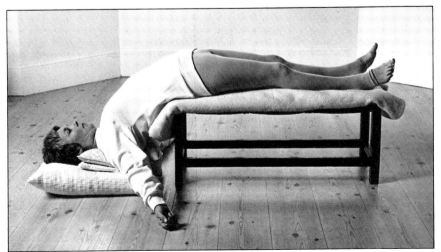

·BANISHING·DEPRESSION·

When you are depressed, you tend to stand with your chest caved in, your shoulders drooping and your head heavy. This posture makes it difficult to look up and face the world, especially as tension builds up in your upper shoulders. Simple stretches that counteract this postural tendency can make you feel better, whether you have been feeling miserable for a short or a long time. However, if your depression is long-standing, it is essential to carry out this programme at least once every day.

1 Shoulders

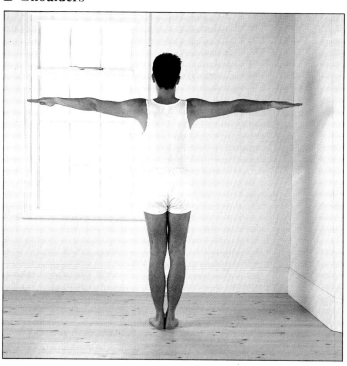
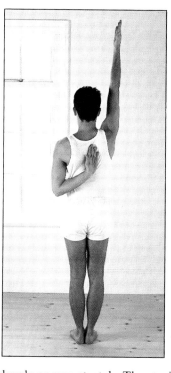

Stand straight and stretch tall. Take your arms out to the side and stretch away from your body (above). Then do the third stretch on p. 103 (above right). Look up and breathe deeply as you stretch. The straighter you stand the easier it will be to catch your hands. Repeat this stretch on each side at least twice.

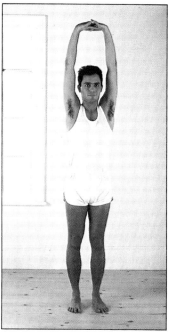

2 Straight

Link your fingers together and turn your palms out. Take your arms up above your head and stretch up as tall as you can. Hold for a few seconds and repeat, with fingers linked the other way.

3 Sideways

Extend your spine by doing one of the stretches on pp. 18-21. Be very careful not to bend forwards. As you stretch to the side, open your chest so that you can breathe in deeply.

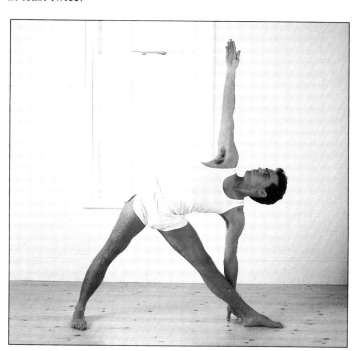

4 Wide and strong

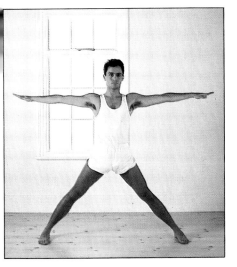 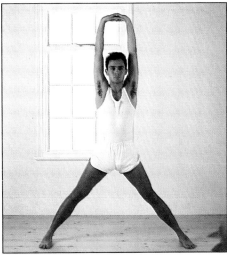 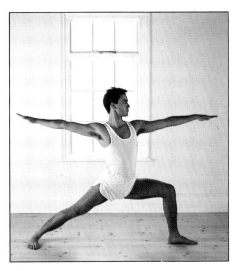

Now do three of the stretches on pp. 22-5, choosing according to your usual level of practice. As you stretch, keep both feet firmly on the ground, spreading out your toes and lifting the arches of your feet. This gives a feeling of stability. Repeat the stretches at least once, alternating sides where this is appropriate.

5 Backwards

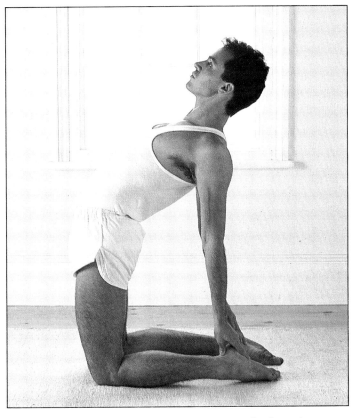

When you have really opened your chest and released your shoulders, kneel on a rug and do one of the stretches on pp. 38-41. Hold the position for a few seconds and then sit on your heels to rest.

6 Relax

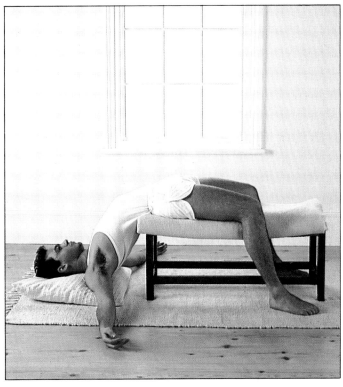

Lie on your back, your trunk raised on a low table, while your head and shoulders are supported on the floor by a cushion. Your knees should be bent, your feet flat on the floor or raised on a very low stool if you prefer. Keep your eyes open and hold for at least 5 minutes. Then slide your back down to the floor and rest before you stand up.

·RENEWING·ENERGY·

You probably do not often express anger and anxiety openly with your body. Instead you are more likely to repress irritation and react to the frustrations that build up in the course of a day by tightening your muscles. If you end a working day full of frustration and aggression, you cannot get going again properly until you have got rid of these negative feelings. This stretch programme will ease the day's tensions and will leave you feeling both relaxed and energetic.

1 Lie down

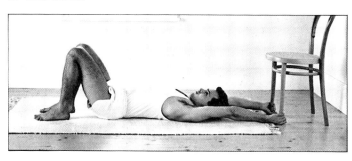

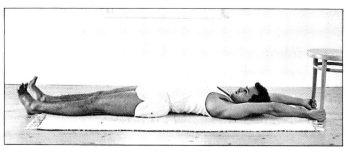

Lie on your back on a rug in front of a chair. Bend your knees, keeping your feet flat on the floor. Reach your arms over your head and grasp the chair legs firmly (top). Extend into your heels as you push the chair away from you (above). Breathe deeply and slowly, then let go of the chair and rest on the floor for a second or two. Repeat once or twice.

2 Legs raised

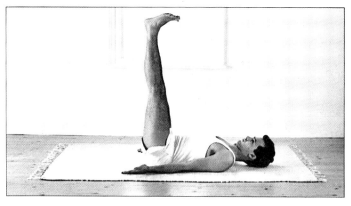

Let go of the chair. Bring your arms down by your sides and bend your knees, sinking your pelvis into the floor. Without arching your back raise your legs over your waist and then straighten them. Hold for a few seconds before bending your knees and bringing your legs down.

3 On your side

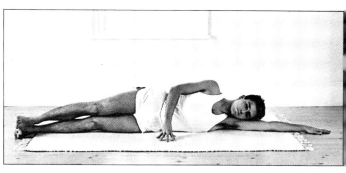

Next bring your legs down and turn on to your left side. Stretch out your left arm and extend the whole of the left side of your body from heel to fingertips.

4 On your side

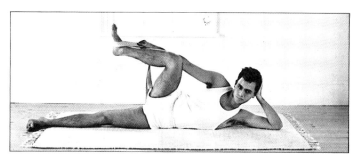

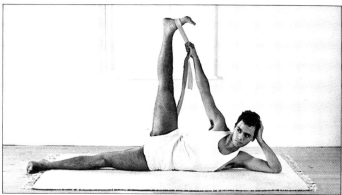

Support your head with your left hand, loop a belt round your right foot and hold on to it, keeping your right knee bent (top). Then straighten your knee and raise your right leg (above). Hold for a few seconds before taking your leg down again. If you find it hard to keep your body in line, practise against a wall. Roll over and repeat steps 3 and 4 on the other side.

5 On all fours

Now turn on to your front and kneel on all fours, your hands and feet body width apart (right). Breathing out, straighten your legs and raise your bottom as high as you can, feet on tiptoe (far right). Keeping your spine and legs stretched, take your heels down towards the floor (below right). Keep your chest open and your neck relaxed to get rid of stiffness in your upper shoulders. Hold for a few seconds before returning to all fours.

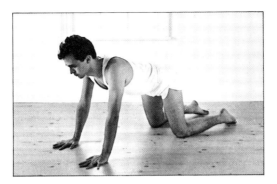

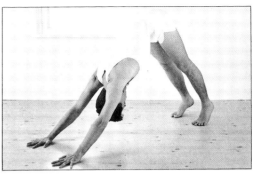

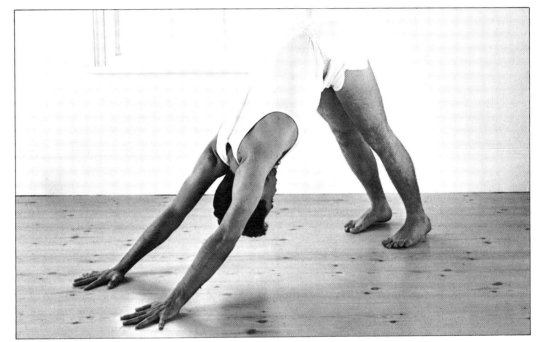

6 Reach out

Stand straight and stretch up through your spine. Finish the sequence by doing one sideways stretch (below) and one wide and strong stretch (below right) from pp. 18-25.

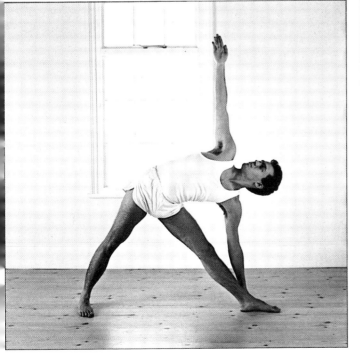

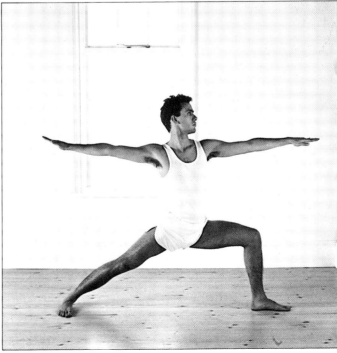

·RECOVERING·FROM·A·JOURNEY·

Travelling often involves sitting in cramped conditions for long periods of time, whether in a car, train or plane. After being confined in a small space for hours on end you are unlikely to relax easily when the journey is over. The further tensions caused by driving in heavy traffic or hanging around at airports make unwinding even more difficult. This programme will relieve travel-related stress and can be done as soon as your journey is over.

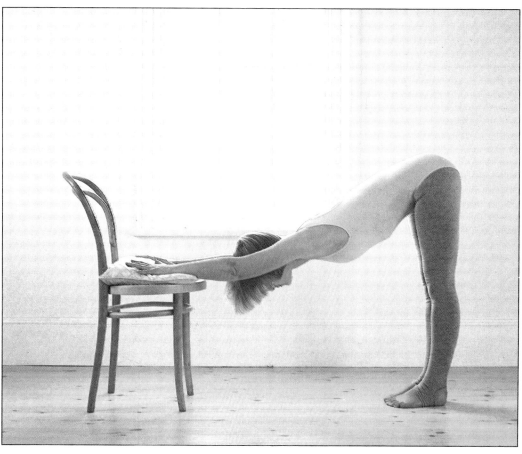

1 Forwards

Stand near a chair and do the first forwards stretch described on p. 32. Bend from your hips, keeping your legs straight. Concentrate on reaching forwards and stretching your shoulders and the backs of your legs. Take your hands down only as far as you can manage without curving your back. Each time you breathe out try to take your chest a little nearer the floor. Hold for up to 1 minute.

2 Twist

Now kneel down on a rug with your knees together and sit on your heels. Interlocking your fingers, breathe out as you stretch your arms above your head, turning your palms upwards (right). Take a few breaths before bringing your arms down. On the next out-breath, twist round as far as step 3 of the basic stretch on p. 34, keeping your shoulders relaxed (far right). Hold for a few seconds before stretching up and twisting round to the other side, maintaining the lift in your spine.

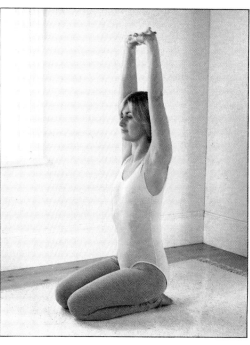

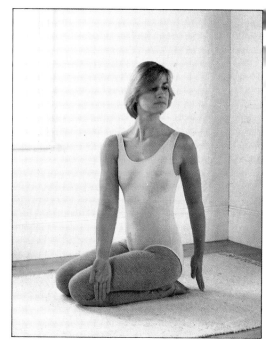

3 Straight

With your knees still together, take your feet apart and sit between your heels (right). (If you are stiff and find this difficult, put a cushion under your buttocks.) Take your hands behind your back and link your fingers (far right). Sitting straight, let your shoulders relax and your hands drop down towards the floor while you open your chest and breathe deeply. Hold for up to 5 minutes.

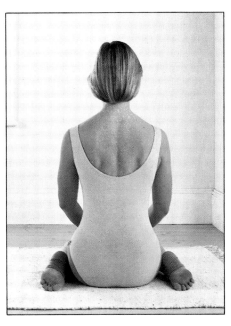
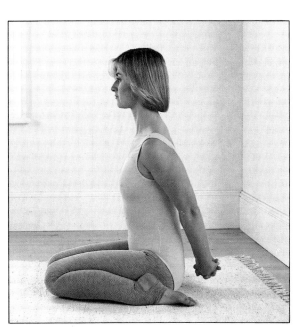

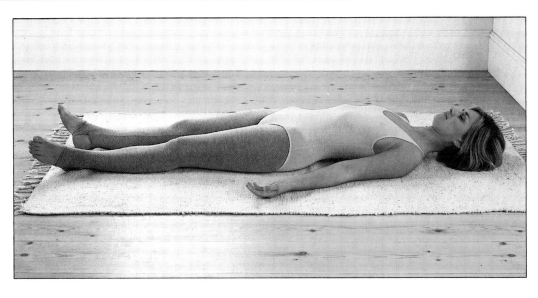

4 Backwards

If you are comfortable sitting between your heels, you can lie back on the floor and stretch the front of your thighs. If your front thigh muscles are very tight – perhaps because you have been walking, cycling or ski-ing – you will be more comfortable lying on a large cushion. Ten minutes in this position is extremely relaxing.
Caution: If you have a history of knee problems, do the relaxation position at the top of p. 53 with your body raised on cushions instead.

5 Relax

Finally lie on a rug on the floor and relax as described on pp. 50-1. Concentrate on making your out-breath long and slow, easing tension in your shoulders and hips. Stay in this position for at least 10 to 15 minutes.

·CALMING·DOWN·

There are some days when the telephone never stops, when home or office seem to demand reserves from you that you do not possess. By the end of such a day you may feel exhausted yet unable to calm down. Your mind is so active that you cannot relax at once, while your body is tired and tight with fatigue so that deep breathing is useless. This programme will help your muscles to relax and your mind to slow down. Gradually you will begin to breathe quietly and deeply.

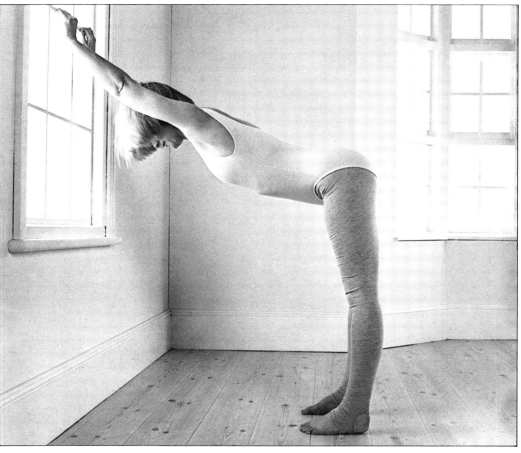

1 Up and forwards

Stand with your feet 15cm (6in) apart. Stretch up and forwards until your hands are resting on a high shelf or window sash. Breathe out and feel your spine stretch from your tailbone towards your head. Continue to breathe slowly and after each out-breath feel the tension ease in your shoulders and upper back. Hold for up to 1 minute.

2 Straight

Now stand straight. Link your fingers together, palms out, and as you breathe in extend your arms to shoulder level. As you breathe out, take them up above your head. Breathe deeply, maintain the stretch in your spine (right). Keep your feet firmly planted on the floor, toes spread out, and feel yourself stretch very tall. Hold for a few seconds. Breathing out, let your arms drop and relax your shoulders (far right). Stand straight and breathe deeply for a minute or two without straining.

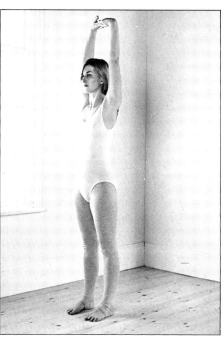

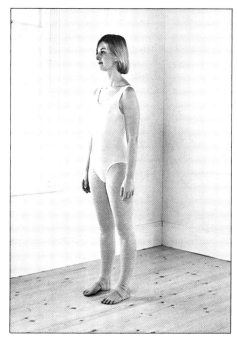

3 On all fours

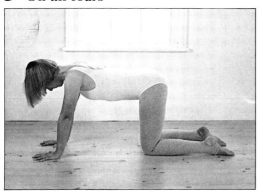

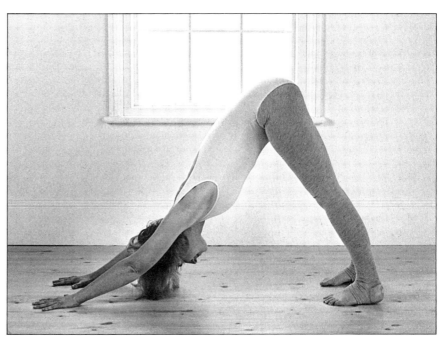

Now kneel on all fours (above). On an out-breath, straighten your legs and take your hips back and up, keeping your back straight. Then take your heels down to the floor (right). Hold for up to 30 seconds, then come back on all fours.

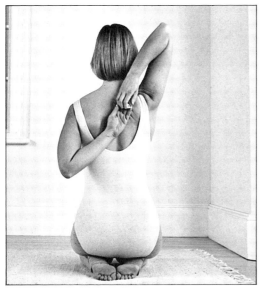

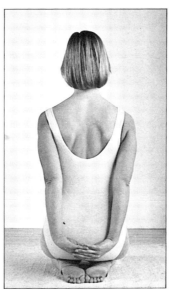

4 Shoulders

Next sit on your heels on a rug, with your knees together. Dropping your shoulders, stretch one arm up and bring the other up behind your back (far left). On an out-breath, catch your hands as shown on p. 103. Do not drop your head forwards, but extend the base of your skull towards the ceiling. Focus your attention on your breath for a few seconds. Then release your hands and change them round. Afterwards, sit quietly on your heels for a minute or two with your shoulders relaxed and your eyes closed, keeping your spine straight and clasping your hands behind you (left). This will relax tight muscles in your neck. If you are still exhausted, repeat two or three times.

5 Relax

Finally lie on a rug on the floor and relax as described on pp. 50-1. Make your out-breath long and slow, easing tension in your shoulders and hips. Stay in this position for at least 10 to 15 minutes.

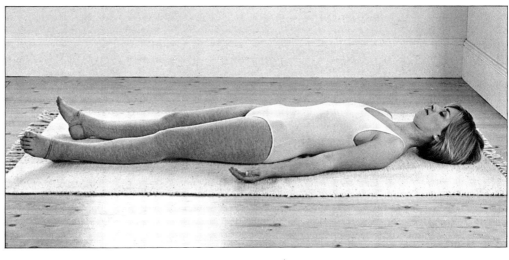

·GETTING·TO·SLEEP·

When you cannot sleep your mind stays active, while your body becomes more and more tense as you toss and turn. This programme will help. Do the whole sequence just before you go to bed. If insomnia is a recurrent problem, doing a regular daily stretch programme will help (see pp. 58-73). Caution: You should avoid stretching forwards if you have a slipped disc or acute back problem.

1 Forwards and sideways

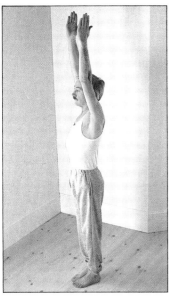 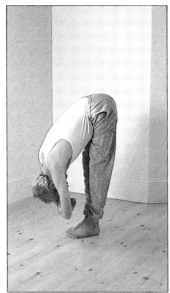 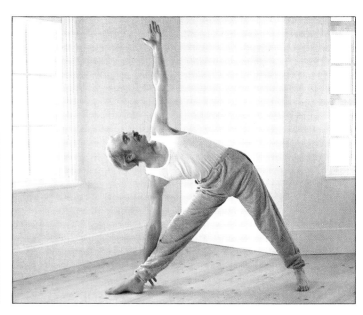

Breathing in, stand tall and stretch your arms above your head (above left). Breathing out, fold your arms and bend forwards from your hips (above centre). Breathe normally for a few seconds, stand straight and then do the basic sideways stretch on pp. 18-19, breathing out (above right). Hold for a few seconds, then repeat on the other side.

2 Forwards and sideways

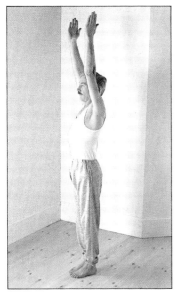 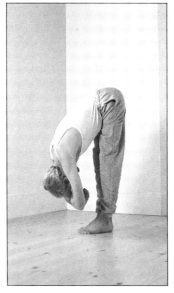 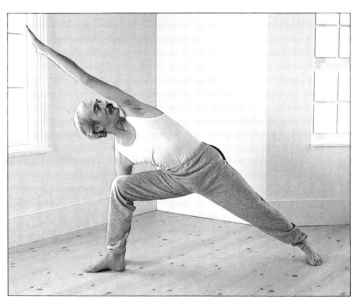

Breathing in, stand tall and stretch your arms above your head (left). Breathing out, fold your arms and bend forwards from your hips (centre). Breathe normally for a few seconds, stand straight and stretch sideways again, doing a more advanced stretch if you can (right). Breathe out as you stretch. Hold for a few seconds, then come up and repeat on the other side.

3 Forwards

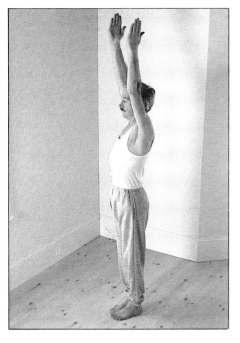 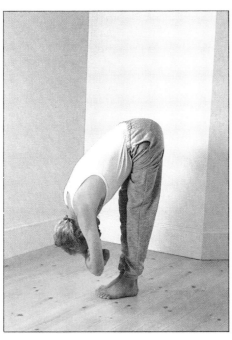

Breathing in, stand tall and stretch your arms above your head (above left). Breathing out, fold your arms and bend forwards from your hips (above centre). Spend at least 1 minute in this position, breathing quietly.

4 Upside down

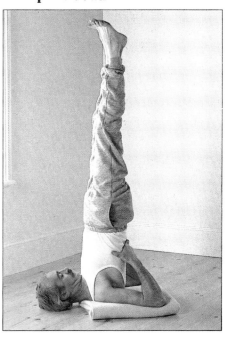

Now do the basic stretch on pp. 42-3 and try to stay in this position for a few minutes. Come down slowly and carefully.

5 Relax

Sit on some cushions and stretch your trunk along your legs, keeping them straight. Let yourself relax into this position and go to bed when you feel sleepy. Caution: If you have a back problem, use an alternative position from pp. 52-3.

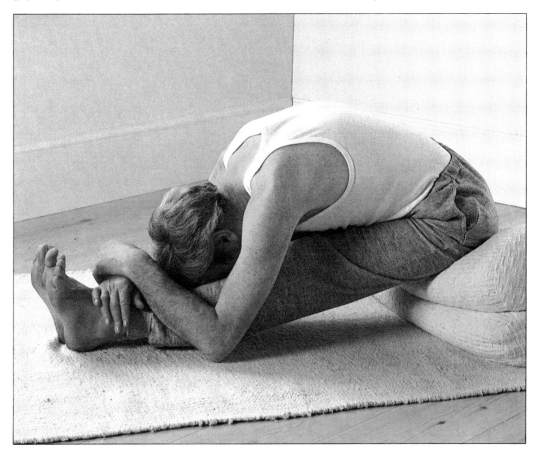

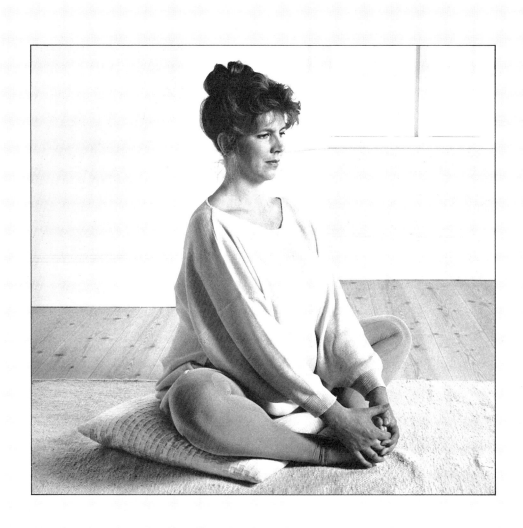

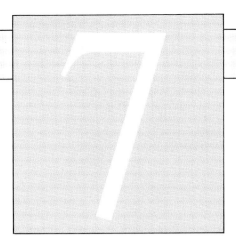

·HAVING·A·BABY·

I f you are already used to practising stretch when you become pregnant, you have a head start, as you will understand the benefit of good posture and a balanced programme of exercise and relaxation. By toning your muscles and opening up your pelvic area, stretching will help to prepare you for birth. It may also help to relieve backache and other minor discomforts. As the baby grows larger, you should find it easy to adapt your normal daily routine, using whichever positions for relaxation you find most comfortable.

If you are starting stretch in pregnancy for the first time, your naturally increased awareness of your body will be a great help. Remember to go slowly and read Chapter One, so that you understand the stretches before you start to practise. During pregnancy even women who usually find it difficult to slow down and concentrate as they stretch and relax find a new sense of harmony with their bodies. Relaxation at this time is essential. It will bring an increased awareness of yourself and your baby, it will help you to cope with your changes of mood and, during labour, it will help you to rest calmly between contractions. By practising control over the rhythm of your breath you will also be preparing yourself for labour. Breathing can help you to feel in control of your body even when contractions are at their strongest.

Birth is not a test to be undergone and passed with top marks; neither is it an end in itself. To see it in this way is to risk disappointment. You may prepare yourself for a particular type of birth and then feel bitterly let down if the reality proves different. Above all, try to be as open-minded as you can about labour and the birth itself. Even if events do not match your expectations, if you exercise in pregnancy your body will be fit, well prepared and better able to cope with the demands of labour and birth. Pages 130-35 suggest a stretch routine suitable for all stages of pregnancy, whether or not you have practised stretch before. On pages 136-37 there is some information about positions that you might find helpful in labour and finally, on pages 138-43, there is a routine for the first six weeks after the birth, after which time you can return to a beginners' or basic stretch programme. If you are in any doubt about your suitability for any of the stretches in this chapter, take medical advice.

·STRETCH·IN·PREGNANCY·

For the most part you can stretch during pregnancy as you would normally, apart from certain modifications described in the instructions for the individual stretches. There are a few specific points to bear in mind:

1 Do not jump your feet into place for the standing stretches; move smoothly into position.
2 Breathe deeply as you stretch. Make real use of your breathing as you move into the positions.
3 You may find that holding a position for the usual length of time becomes a strain. If so, do each movement briefly but repeat it several times.
4 Feel that each stretch gives your baby more space inside you.
5 Always make sure you are lifting up and stretching away from your pelvic floor (see below) as you move.
6 Do not lie flat on your back in late pregnancy, as the baby may press against one of your major blood vessels in this position, depriving itself of oxygen or making you feel faint.

Relaxation

During the first few months of pregnancy you can continue to relax as usual, using the techniques described in the chapter on relaxation (see pages 48-57). As the birth of your baby approaches, try to give a little more time to relaxation with deep breathing (see pages 54-7), prolonging only every third or fourth out-breath.

Pelvic-floor muscles

The muscles of your pelvic floor are the ones that surround the anus and the vagina. You can feel them tightening if you try to stop urinating in mid-flow. During pregnancy you should practise tightening and releasing these muscles several times every day – tighten them as you breathe in and let go as you breathe out. Exercising these muscles is very important: if they become slack, sexual intercourse may become less pleasurable and, in the long term, other problems such as incontinence may result. You can do pelvic-floor

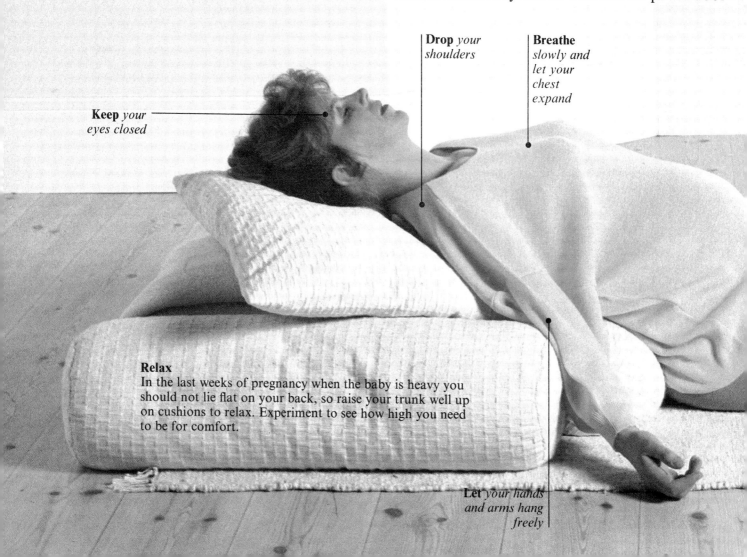

Keep *your eyes closed*

Drop *your shoulders*

Breathe *slowly and let your chest expand*

Relax
In the last weeks of pregnancy when the baby is heavy you should not lie flat on your back, so raise your trunk well up on cushions to relax. Experiment to see how high you need to be for comfort.

Let *your hands and arms hang freely*

exercises while carrying on with all sorts of
ordinary daily activities, including stretch. At
first practise when standing straight. As you gain
awareness and control of the muscles, you will
feel strong and able to control the pelvic floor as
you stretch in all directions. In labour this awareness will help you give birth with control.

Standing straight

As the baby grows, its weight pulls you forwards
and the top of your spine bends back to compensate. If you stand badly out of alignment, the added
weight of the baby puts excessive strain on the
structure of your body. Instead of the spine and
pelvis providing the correct support, the strain will
be taken by ligaments and muscles not intended
for the job. If you are sway-backed to start with
(see page 93), the curve at the back of your waist will
increase, putting a further strain on the muscles
of your lower back and giving rise to backache.

Think about how you stand, not just when you
are practising stretch but in everyday life. If you
tend to be sway-backed and suffer from backache,
practise the straight stretch (right) followed by
relaxation (below) more than once a day.

Straight

Stand against the edge of a door, keeping your heels down.
The backs of your heels, your lower back and the back of
your head should touch the door. Then stretch your arms up
so that they hold the top of the door (loop a belt over the
top if the door is too high). Breathe deeply, and enjoy
stretching tall. Hold for a few seconds, then take your arms
down and stand as before, breathing deeply.

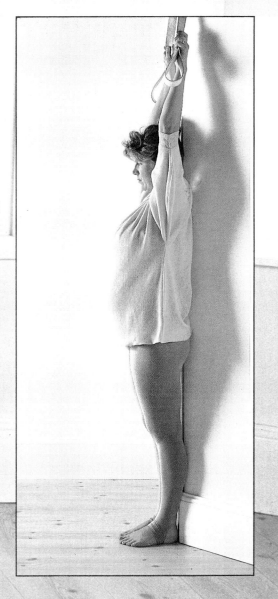

Make sure
*your feet
and toes are
relaxed*

·STRETCH·IN·PREGNANCY·

The weight of the baby is going to pull you forwards as you stretch sideways, making it hard to extend fully. Using a wall for guidance will make the correct stretch easier to feel. Do not lean on the wall; just be aware of it behind you, keeping you in line.

As you get heavier, you may find the basic stretches quite difficult, especially the wide and strong position with hips down and knee bent. If at any time you feel uncomfortable in a position, or as if you are constricting your baby, do a simple "less stretch" movement instead of a basic stretch.

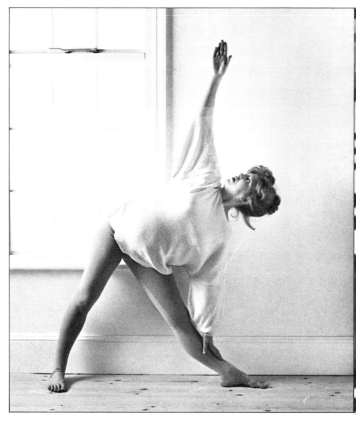

Sideways (right)
Standing with a wall behind you, follow the instructions on pp. 18-19. The heel of your back foot should touch the wall, with your out-turned foot slightly in front of it. As you reach sideways, feel both shoulders brush the wall; do not let yourself bend forwards. Hold for a few seconds. Breathe in, come up and repeat on the other side.

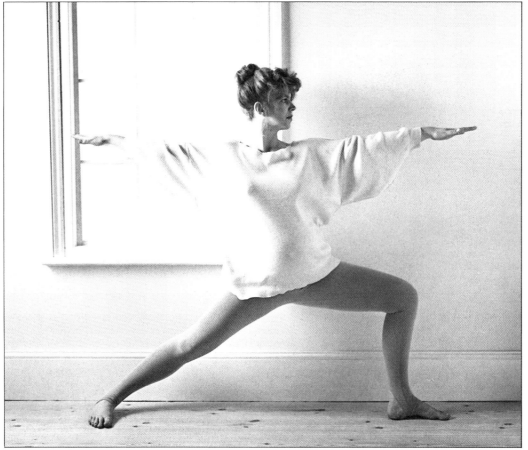

Wide and strong
With a wall behind you for guidance, follow the instructions on pp. 22-3. Keep the heel of your back foot in contact with the wall, while your out-turned foot is a little in front of it. Take your hips down as far as you comfortably can, lifting up from your pelvic floor as you stretch up and out. Hold for a few seconds, then breathe in and come up. Repeat on the other side.

If you have practised the basic back to the centre stretch regularly from the very beginning of pregnancy, you should not find balancing on one leg a problem even in the last weeks. However, towards the end of pregnancy, you may prefer to stand within reach of a wall, so that you can steady yourself with one hand as you use the other to get yourself into position. Make use of the feeling of calmness that you should experience to focus your whole attention on your growing baby.

The forwards stretch shown below is especially good for pregnancy because your arms are supported, making it easy to stretch and relax at the same time. With your forearms taking some of your body weight, you can concentrate on stretching the backs of your thighs to achieve the correct rotation of the pelvis.

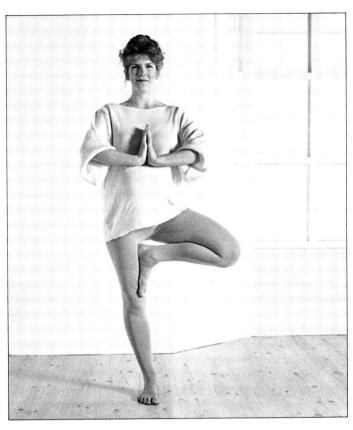

Back to the centre (right)
Follow the instructions on pp. 26-7, steadying yourself against a wall with one hand if you find it hard to balance on one leg. Wait until you feel securely balanced before aligning your fingers and pressing your palms together evenly. Hold for a few seconds, breathe in and take your foot down. Repeat on the other side.

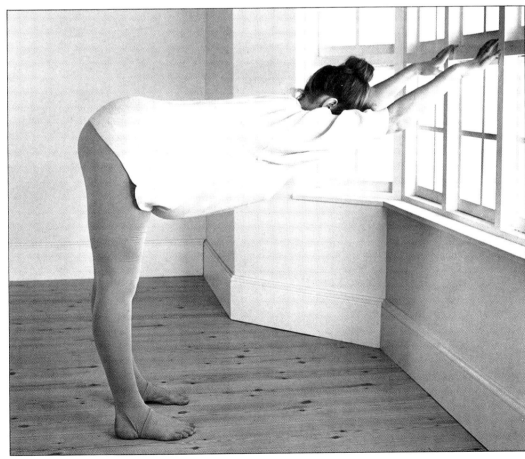

Forwards
Stretch forwards as far as your back thigh muscles (hamstrings) will allow you to extend, following the instructions on p. 32. If the backs of your legs feel tight, reach out to a point high on a wall or window; if you are more supple, you can reach down as far as a chair seat. Lift up from your pelvic floor as you stretch, feeling the extra room for your baby as your spine extends. Hold for up to 30 seconds, then come up breathing in.

·STRETCH·IN·PREGNANCY·

There are no upside down positions illustrated on these pages because many women find stretching upside down uncomfortable in pregnancy and stop doing it. As with all the stretches, this is a matter for your common sense. If you wish to continue stretching upside down in pregnancy, seek the advice of an experienced teacher. If you did not do any stretch before you became pregnant, leave the upside down positions until after the birth.

In any case, whether or not you stretch upside down after the twist and backwards stretch, you should finish your practice with the two back to the centre movements on the opposite page. Both these positions loosen stiffness in the pelvis and help prepare you for the birth of your baby.

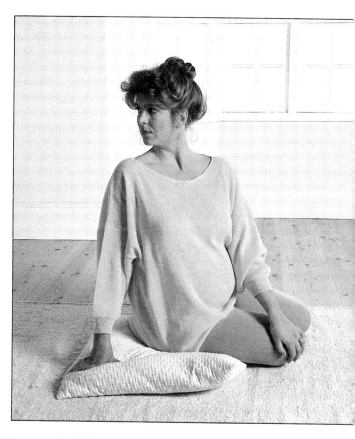

Twist (right)
Sitting on a cushion, follow the instructions for the basic stretch on pp. 34-5. Feel that you are giving your baby plenty of space by stretching up as you turn, and keep the fingertips of your right hand on the cushion or floor to help you maintain the upward lift. Hold your spine in a straight line, with the back of your head directly above the back of your hips. Stay in the position for a few seconds, breathe in and come up. Repeat on the other side.

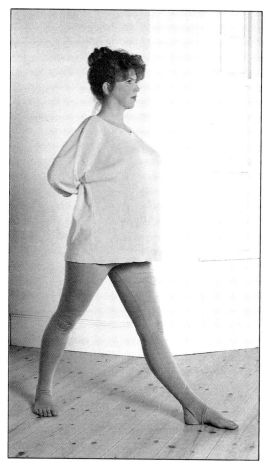

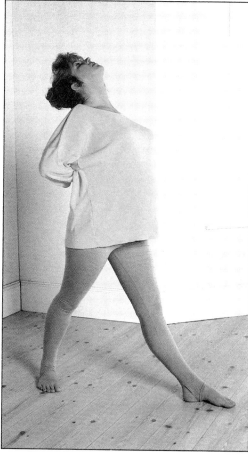

Backwards
Take your feet 1m (3ft) apart. Turn your right foot slightly in and your left leg out, aligning your left heel with your right arch. Then turn your whole trunk to the left. Take your arms behind you and turn your hands up, fingers pointing upwards and palms together. Pressing your palms against each other, take your elbows back (far left).

Stretch up, breathing in. Then breathe out and bend back. Your lower spine should extend as you stretch up, and your upper back should lift and stretch backwards as you continue to press your hands together (left). Hold for a few seconds, breathe in and come back to vertical. Take two or three deep breaths and repeat on the other side.

Note: If you are unable to take your hands up behind your back, catch your elbows behind your waist instead.

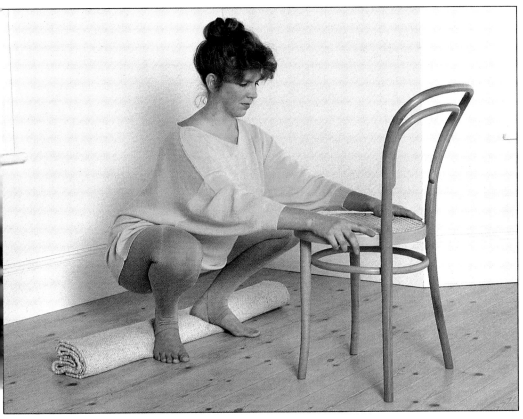

Back to the centre
Stand facing a chair, your
feet about 30cm (1ft) apart.
Bending at your hips and
knees, squat down, holding
the chair to steady yourself.
Try to keep your feet flat on
the floor; if this is impossible, put a folded blanket
under your heels. Press your
heels down and open out
your knees, keeping your
back straight. Breathe
quietly and hold for as long
as you comfortably can.
When you can stay in this
position for 30 seconds and
keep your balance, you can
dispense with the chair.
(This is a good position for
practising pelvic-floor
exercises – see p. 130.)

Back to the centre
Follow the instructions on
p. 29, putting a cushion under
your buttocks if your hip
joints are not flexible or if
your lower back tends to
collapse. Do the stretch more
than once a day if you can,
holding it for a few
seconds longer each time
you practise.
   Although this position is
considered difficult, you may
find it easier than you
imagine, because the joints
of the pelvis become more
mobile in pregnancy.

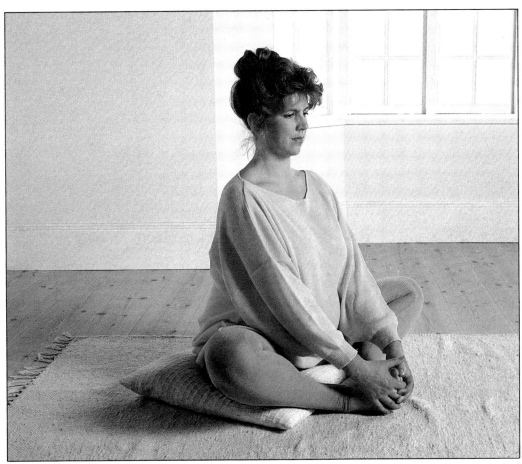

·POSITIONS·FOR·LABOUR·

Stretching and relaxing during pregnancy will naturally extend into preparation for labour. By the time your baby is ready to be born you should have a good understanding of your body, know how to relax and be in tune with your breathing.

Animals automatically find the most comfortable and convenient way in which to deliver their young, and women need to be free to do the same during labour. Over the years various considerations – including fashion and the convenience of medical attendants – have dictated the positions and movements of mothers during childbirth. By restricting women to unsuitable positions, certain techniques have even added to the distress they were intended to alleviate.

However, recently it has been suggested that allowing and encouraging women to be active in labour has not only made deliveries quicker and less painful but has also reduced the need for medical intervention.

Labour is a time when you need to feel free and uninhibited. Because social custom usually restricts you to certain forms of behaviour, you may not be used to being spontaneous in your movements. It is therefore a good idea during pregnancy to practise various positions that you might find helpful in labour and to imagine how you might want to behave during intense contractions. You may also find some of the positions illustrated relaxing when you want to rest in the last few weeks, as it can be hard to get comfortable when the baby is large.

The best positions in labour are those where the pull of gravity assists the delivery of the baby. Sitting back on your tailbone, for instance, is not a good position, because your tailbone impedes the passage of the baby; lying flat on your back is not good either, because you have to push against gravity and the baby may become short of oxygen. In the first stage you should move around as much as you are able to, adopting many different positions; as the birth draws near and you find it harder to move around, try to settle in a position where the pelvis is free to open naturally.

Forwards (left)
Try stretching up and forwards, feet apart. Rest comfortably against a wall or a window and cradle your head in your arms (if you prefer you could stretch your arms out).

Sitting (below)
Sit astride a straight-backed chair and rest your head on your arms supported by cushions, your feet flat on the floor (you can put a cushion on the chair seat if you like).

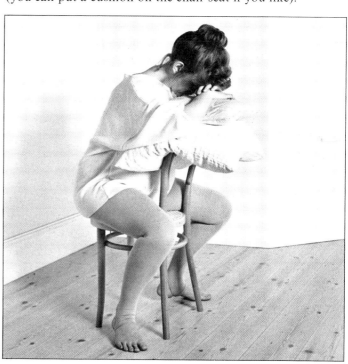

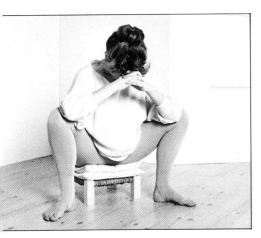

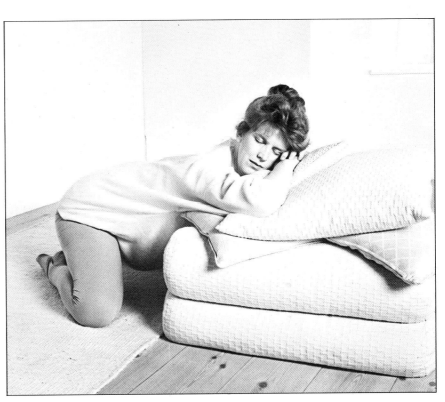

Squatting (above)
Lower yourself into the squatting position, with some cushions on a low stool under your buttocks for support. With your feet flat on the floor, rest your elbows on your knees and your head on your hands.

Kneeling on to cushions (right)
Kneel with your knees wide apart, resting your head and arms on a pile of cushions.

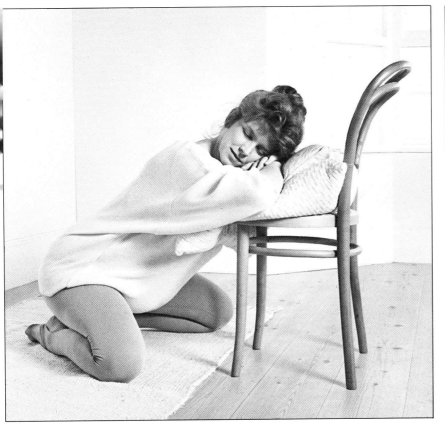

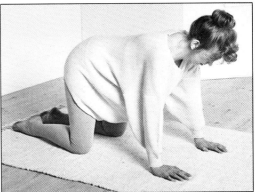

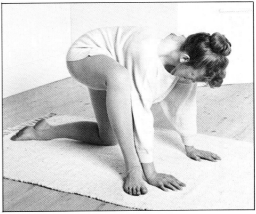

Kneeling on to a chair
Have your knees wide apart and kneel with your head and arms resting on a chair seat, using cushions for support. By keeping your body vertical, this can help to speed up labour.

On all fours
Go on to all fours, letting your spine extend, rocking if this is helpful (top). You may prefer the position with one knee bent (above).

·AFTER·THE·BIRTH·

Most new mothers are unprepared for the tiredness of the first few days – and often weeks – after the birth. Giving birth takes all your strength, both physical and emotional. You and your baby also need time to adapt to life as two separate people. For a few weeks at least try to avoid too many outside pressures; adjust to your new rhythm at your own pace.

With a small baby, your daily routine will be completely different. You may find it very difficult to give time to stretching and relaxation, especially if you have other children already. In fact, stretch will repay you for your time with energy and strength. If you were very fit and active before the birth, practising stretch regularly, the post-natal exercises will come more easily. You will quickly regain your shape and fitness, as day by day you re-tone your muscles.

Deliveries vary, so how soon you can do a particular stretch will depend to some extent on you. If at first some of the stretches don't feel right – for instance because you have stitches that pull –

just do the simpler first movements for a few extra days, repeating them often if you wish. Use your common sense, and introduce new movements when you feel ready. If you have had a Caesarean delivery, however, you *must* consult your obstetrician before you start any form of exercise.

The following pages suggest a programme of exercises for the first six weeks or so after you have had your baby. Each of the first five weeks introduces some new movements into a suggested daily routine, and these new movements are picked out by a coloured border. When the instructions to the stretches refer to a basic stretch from Chapter One, you should substitute a "less stretch" movement if this is more suited to your usual stretch level. At the end of six weeks, you can start doing a complete beginners' or basic programme, continuing to include shoulder stretches and pelvic-floor exercises. If you were doing a more advanced programme before you became pregnant, you can return to it three months after the birth.

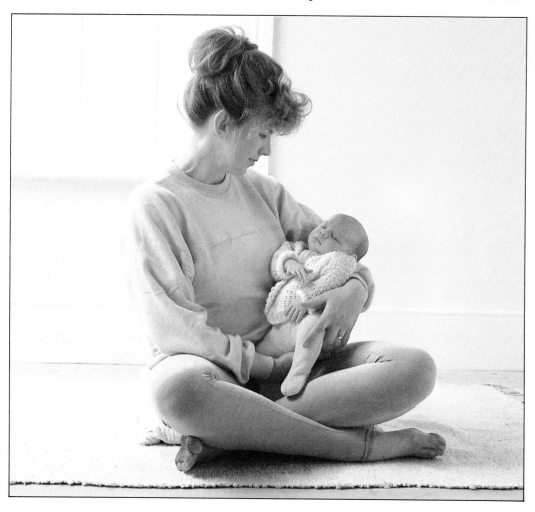

Mother and child
Let the time you can give to stretching and relaxation reward you with renewed energy, so that you can truly enjoy your new baby in the very first weeks of her life.

· WEEK · ONE ·

Straight

Lie flat on your back on a
rug with your knees bent
and your arms stretched
above your head (above
right). Keep the back of your
waist flat on the floor. Slowly
straighten your legs, keeping
your waist extended (below
right). Tighten your stomach
muscles and your pelvic-floor
muscles (see p. 130). Stretch
from your heels to your
fingertips for a few seconds.
Relax and repeat the stretch
several times.

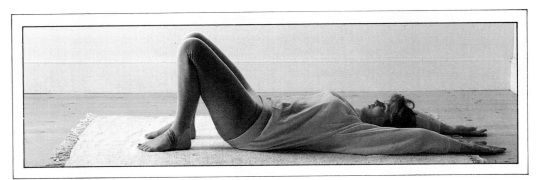

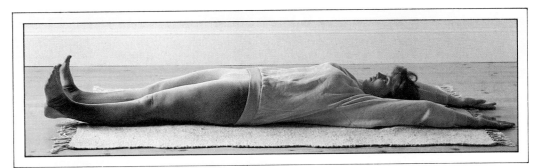

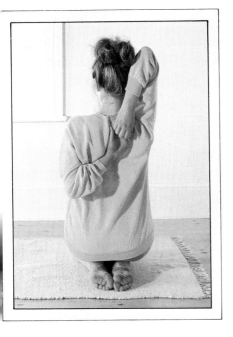

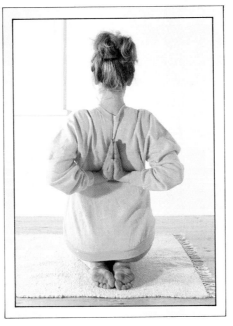

2 Shoulders

Sit on your heels and clasp
your hands behind your back
(far left) as described on p.
103. Hold for a few seconds,
then repeat with your hands
the other way round. Next
fold your hands up behind
your back, palms together
(left). As you take your
elbows back, breathe deeply
and open your chest. Hold
for a few seconds and repeat.

These shoulder stretches
are especially important for
as long as you are feeding
your baby and bending over
her a great deal.

3 Relax

Lie flat on your back on the floor to
relax. If this is uncomfortable, choose
an alternative position from pp. 52-3.
Stay in the position for at least 5 to
10 minutes.

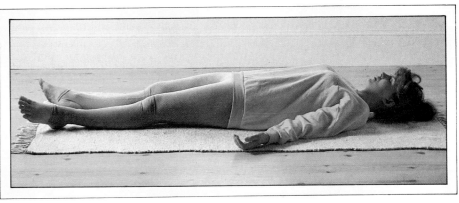

·WEEK·TWO·

1 Straight

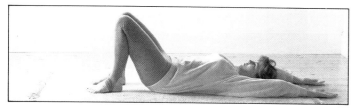

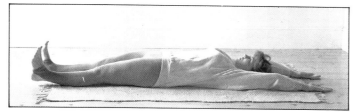

2 Shoulders

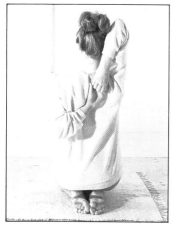 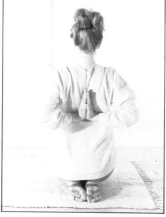

3 Forwards

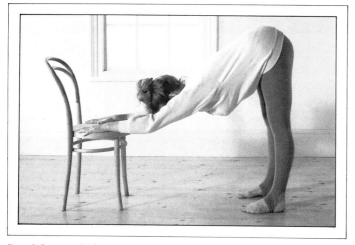

Bend forwards from your hips as shown on p. 32. Breathe deeply, then, at the end of an out-breath, pull your stomach muscles in strongly towards your spine, at the same time squeezing your pelvic-floor muscles. Relax your grip as you breathe in. Take a few deep breaths, repeat and come up.

4 Backwards

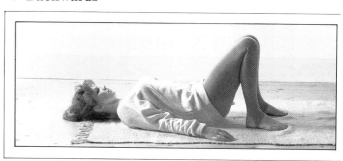

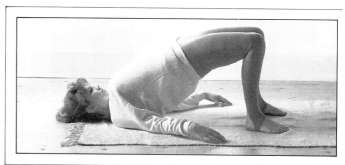

Lie flat on your back on a rug with your knees bent (top). Take a few deep breaths, then lift up your hips on an out-breath, tucking in your tailbone and tightening your buttock muscles (above). Keep your arms on the floor. Hold for a few seconds, breathe in and come down.

5 Back to the centre

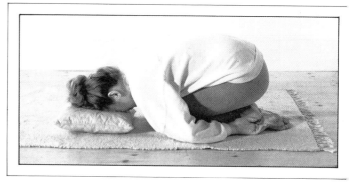

Kneel and bend forwards as shown on p. 28. Keep your buttocks down on your heels and relax your neck and shoulders. Hold for a few seconds, breathe in and come up.

6 Relax

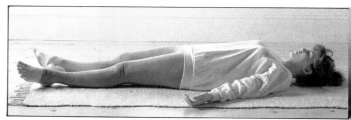

· WEEK · THREE ·

1 Straight

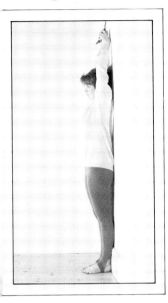

Now you can stand up to stretch tall (left). Use the edge of the door as you did when you were pregnant (see p. 131). Tighten your pelvic-floor muscles and your stomach muscles in the same way as you did when lying flat.

Stay standing straight to do the shoulder stretches from Weeks One and Two (right and far right). Hold each one for a few seconds and repeat several times.

2 Shoulders

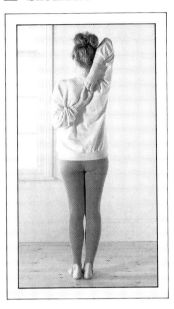
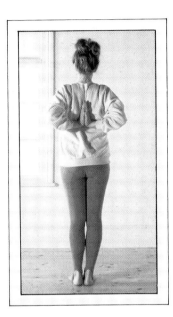

3 Forwards

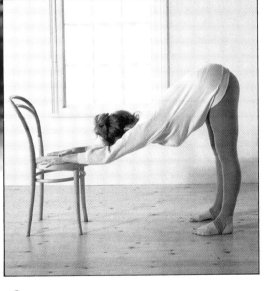

4 Twist

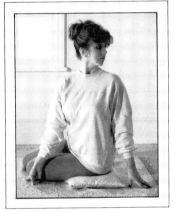

Do the basic twist as described on pp. 34-5. Hold for a few seconds, breathe in and face forwards.

5 Backwards

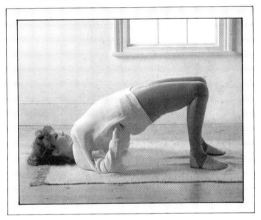

Do the stretch you started in Week Two. If you can lift up your hips high enough, support your back with your hands. Hold for a few seconds, breathe in and come down.

6 Back to the centre

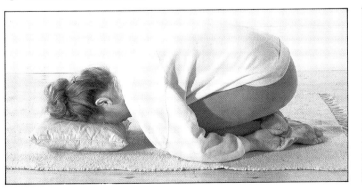

7 Relax

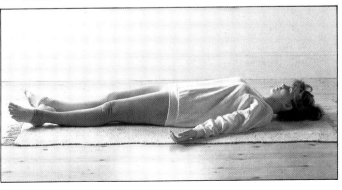

·WEEK·FOUR·

1 Straight

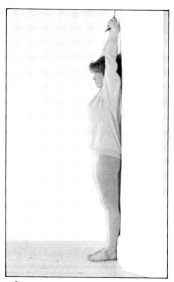

2 Shoulders

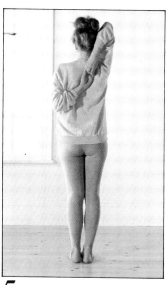

3 Forwards

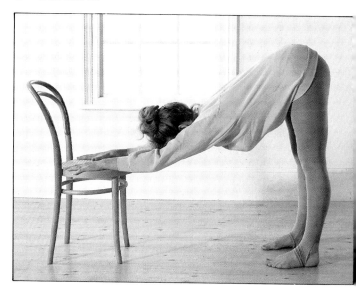

4 Twist

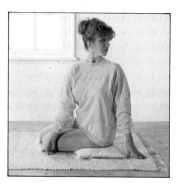

5 Backwards

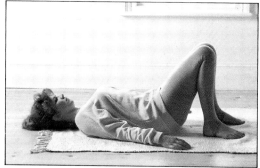

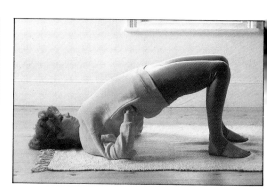

6 Backwards

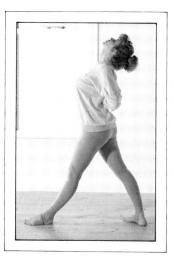

7 Back to the centre

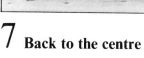

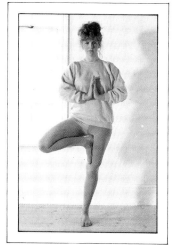

8 Back to the centre

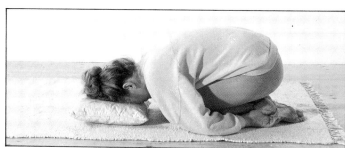

9 Relax

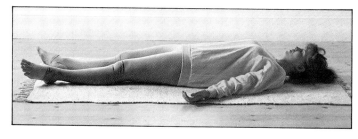

Add the stretch that you did when pregnant (see p. 134). Hold for a few seconds, breathe in and come up.

Do the basic stretch on pp. 26-7. Hold for a few seconds, then repeat standing on the other leg.

· WEEKS · FIVE & SIX ·

1 Straight

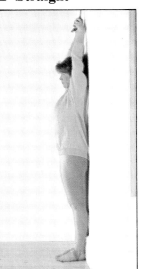

2 Shoulders

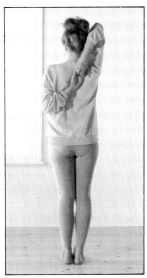

3 Sideways

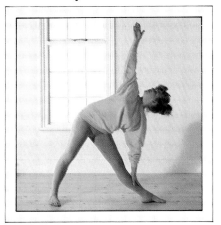

Add the basic stretch on pp. 18-19. Hold for a few seconds. Breathe in, come up and repeat on the other side.

4 Back to the centre

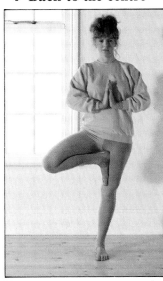

5 Forwards

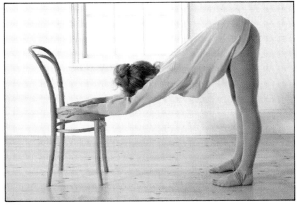

6 Twist

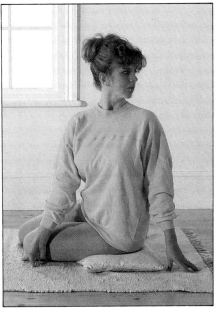

7 Backwards

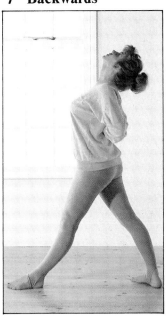

8 Upside down

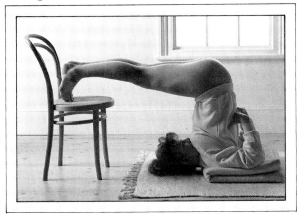

Include the basic position from pp. 42-3. Hold for a few minutes. Then take your feet back on to a chair (see p. 46) for a few seconds. Bend your knees over your head and bring your back gently down.

9 Relax

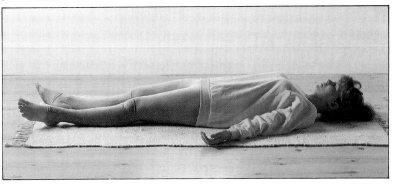

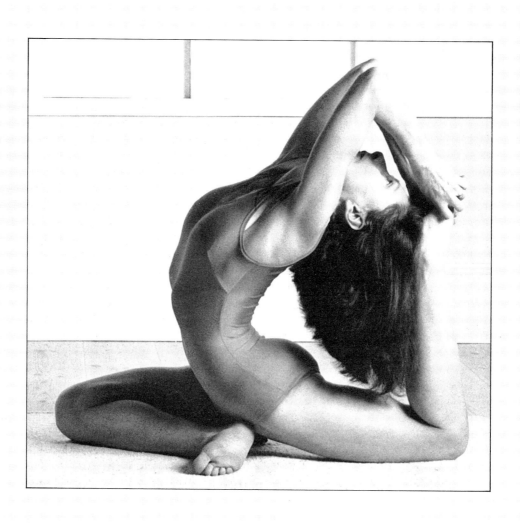

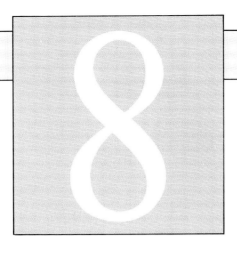

·STRETCH·FURTHER·

The intense stretches described in this chapter are for those who enjoy the freedom of movement that stretching brings, who can do all the other stretches in this book with ease and who would like to stretch further. Although it is possible to practise by yourself without attending classes, it is safer to have some expert guidance. If you want to embark on an advanced stretching programme, the help of an experienced teacher will be invaluable.

The stretches in this chapter are not suitable for inclusion in a twenty-minute daily programme. To extend the body this far with safety, you will need to warm up gradually and take time to relax fully afterwards, however fit and supple you are. A sudden stretch when the body is not prepared can cause injury to muscles or tendons. It is impossible here to give a warm-up routine to suit everyone, as flexibility differs so much from person to person, and everybody needs to warm up in different ways. Working with a good teacher will help you to evolve a warm-up routine and practice to suit your own particular body type.

Advanced stretches have to be part of a regular daily discipline, which takes a lot of time and dedication. It is not safe to do them every now and then when you have a little more time to spare. Were you to stretch in an intense practice just once a week, the following day your body would feel bruised and exhausted instead of free and relaxed. Neither is it sensible to practise the stretches individually, however easy you may find a specific movement. Daily practice is essential, for stretching in this chapter is the culmination of continuous regular practice of the other stretches in this book. These advanced stretches should be part of a weekly routine where daily programmes are adapted, so a different stretch can be practised each day. All the stretches have to be preceded by less intense movements of the same type and followed by counter-movements, upside down stretches and a long period of relaxation.

In order to understand the movements of your own body and the correct action of the stretches, a great deal of time and patience is required in addition to the help of a teacher. Although these are difficult and demanding stretches, which appear somewhat daunting to most people, expert help, time and dedication can bring them within the range of many more people than is generally realized.

· SIDEWAYS ·

The first of these stretches involves an intense sideways stretch in the spine. Your hips stay straight while your spine extends. In the second position you stretch your whole body sideways. As long as you keep your shoulders back correctly, as in the basic sideways stretch, you should find this movement straightforward.

First stretch

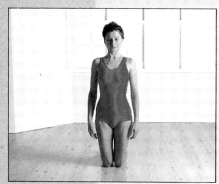

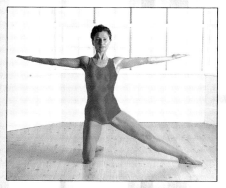

1 Kneel up with your tailbone tucked in and the tops of your feet flat on the floor behind you. Stretch up through your spine.

2 Extend your left leg, keeping the heel of your left foot in line with your right knee. Drop your shoulders and stretch out your arms, palms up.

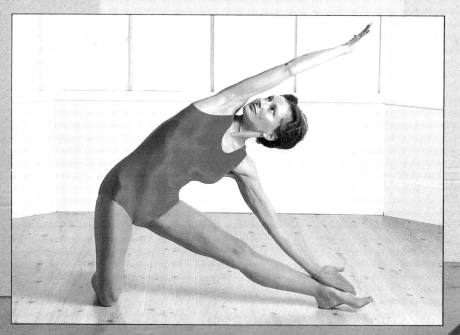

3 Breathing out, extend your trunk to the left, stretching from your hips until the back of your left hand rests on your left foot. Keeping your right thigh vertical, stretch from your lower back, bringing your right arm over your head. Breathe normally for a few seconds, then come up breathing in and repeat on the other side.

Second stretch

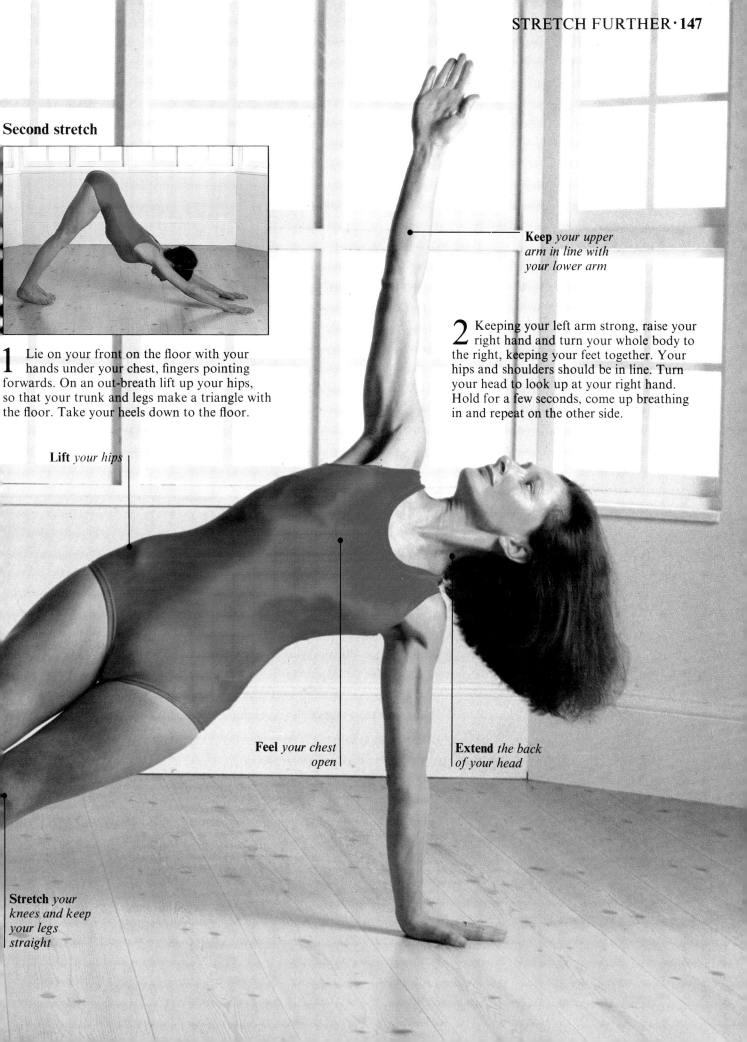

1 Lie on your front on the floor with your hands under your chest, fingers pointing forwards. On an out-breath lift up your hips, so that your trunk and legs make a triangle with the floor. Take your heels down to the floor.

Keep *your upper arm in line with your lower arm*

2 Keeping your left arm strong, raise your right hand and turn your whole body to the right, keeping your feet together. Your hips and shoulders should be in line. Turn your head to look up at your right hand. Hold for a few seconds, come up breathing in and repeat on the other side.

Lift *your hips*

Feel *your chest open*

Extend *the back of your head*

Stretch *your knees and keep your legs straight*

·WIDE & STRONG·

This beautiful position involves an intense stretch in the thigh muscles and requires strong back muscles. The full splits position is best attempted only by experienced students under the guidance of a teacher: practise slowly and never force yourself in any way.

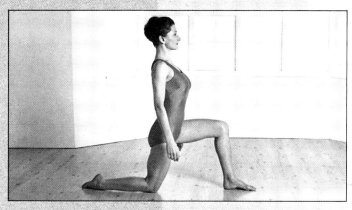

1 Kneel on one knee. Face forwards, keeping your hips straight. Stretch up through your spine, opening your chest as you breathe in.

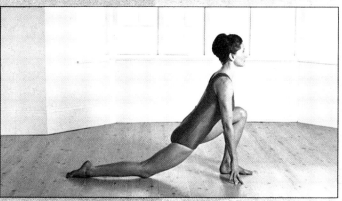

2 On an out-breath bend forwards and put your hands on the floor. Keep your spine stretched from tailbone to head, without tightening your neck or your shoulders.

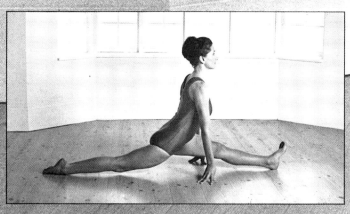

3 Breathe in. As you breathe out again slide your front leg forwards, supporting your weight with your hands. Keep your hips facing forwards as far as possible and let your back leg straighten. Your back knee should face the floor, your front knee the ceiling.

Keep *your back knee facing the floor*

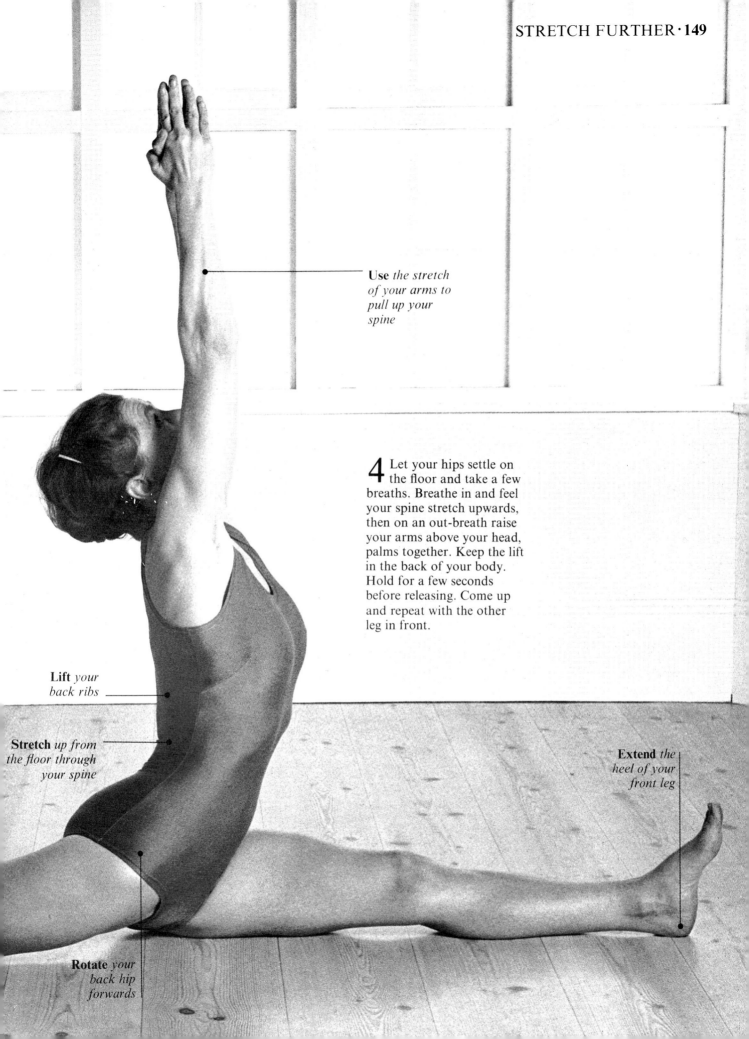

Use *the stretch of your arms to pull up your spine*

4 Let your hips settle on the floor and take a few breaths. Breathe in and feel your spine stretch upwards, then on an out-breath raise your arms above your head, palms together. Keep the lift in the back of your body. Hold for a few seconds before releasing. Come up and repeat with the other leg in front.

Lift *your back ribs*

Stretch *up from the floor through your spine*

Extend *the heel of your front leg*

Rotate *your back hip forwards*

·BACK·TO·THE·CENTRE·

This stretch is a continuation of the "more stretch" position on page 29. You need a flexible back and hips to attempt it. If you should get cramp as a result of bending your spine instead of stretching it, come up and lie flat with knees bent.

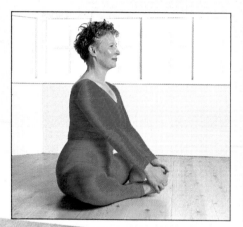

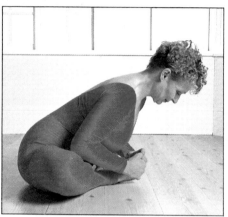

1 Sit with your knees bent, feet together close to your body and your back straight. Keep your shoulders relaxed and let both thighs drop down towards the floor.

2 Holding your feet, breathe out and stretch forwards, extending the whole of the front of your trunk. Continue to drop your thighs towards the floor.

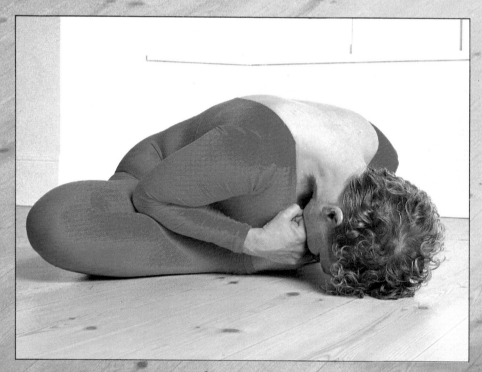

3 Rest your head on the floor. Your whole spine should be stretched and your chest open. Hold the position for two or three breaths, breathe in and come up.

·FORWARDS·

This stretch takes a lot of time and patience, as the insides of your thighs and knees need to extend. Never force or strain, just allow your legs to stretch gradually in the basic and "more stretch" positions (see pages 30-3).

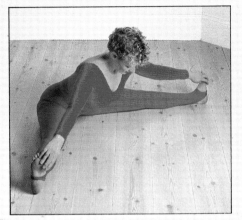

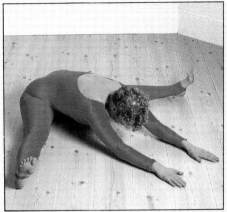

1 Sit with your legs wide apart, so that you are facing the centre between your feet. Extend your heels and straighten your knees. Catch your feet with your hands and feel your lower back move up and in before you go any further.

2 Put your hands in front of you on the floor. Keeping the front of your body extended, stretch forwards, your spine lengthening as you breathe in.

Keep *your buttock bones pressing against the floor*

Extend *your whole spine*

Stretch *your heels strongly*

Relax *the back of your neck*

Stretch *your arms wide and open your chest*

3 As you breathe out, go further forwards and take your hands to your feet. Do not pull forwards with your hands but stretch from your lower spine. On the next out-breath put your head and chest on the floor. Hold for a second or two, breathe in and come up.

·TWIST·

This standing twist demands flexible hips, so that as your upper back turns your chest stays open and unconstricted. You need to turn from the hips without forcing or pushing your shoulders hard against the outside of your knee. At first you will take several breaths as you move into the stretch, but eventually you will be able to do the whole movement on one breath.

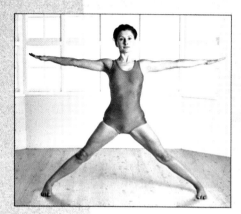 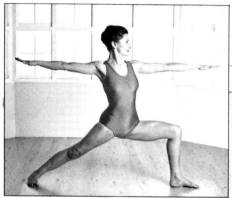 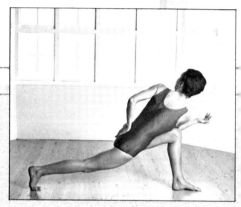

1 Stand tall and straight, stretching up through the curves of your spine. Take your feet wide apart, keeping the stretch in your back. Extend your arms at shoulder level and stretch into your fingertips, the palms of your hands facing the floor.

2 Turn your right foot slightly in and your left leg out, aligning your left heel with the arch of your right foot. Turn your head to the left, as you bend your left knee and take your hips down. Keep the stretch wide and strong.

3 Lift up your right heel and on an out-breath turn your whole trunk to the left. Keep your left thigh parallel to the floor, your knee back. Put your left hand on your hip, then twist around and take your right arm behind your left knee.

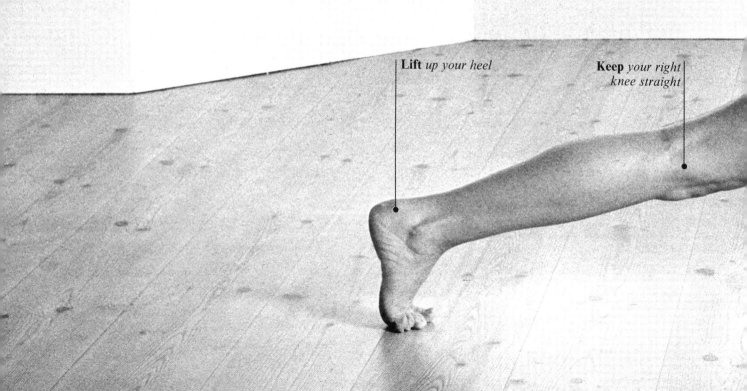

Lift *up your heel*

Keep *your right knee straight*

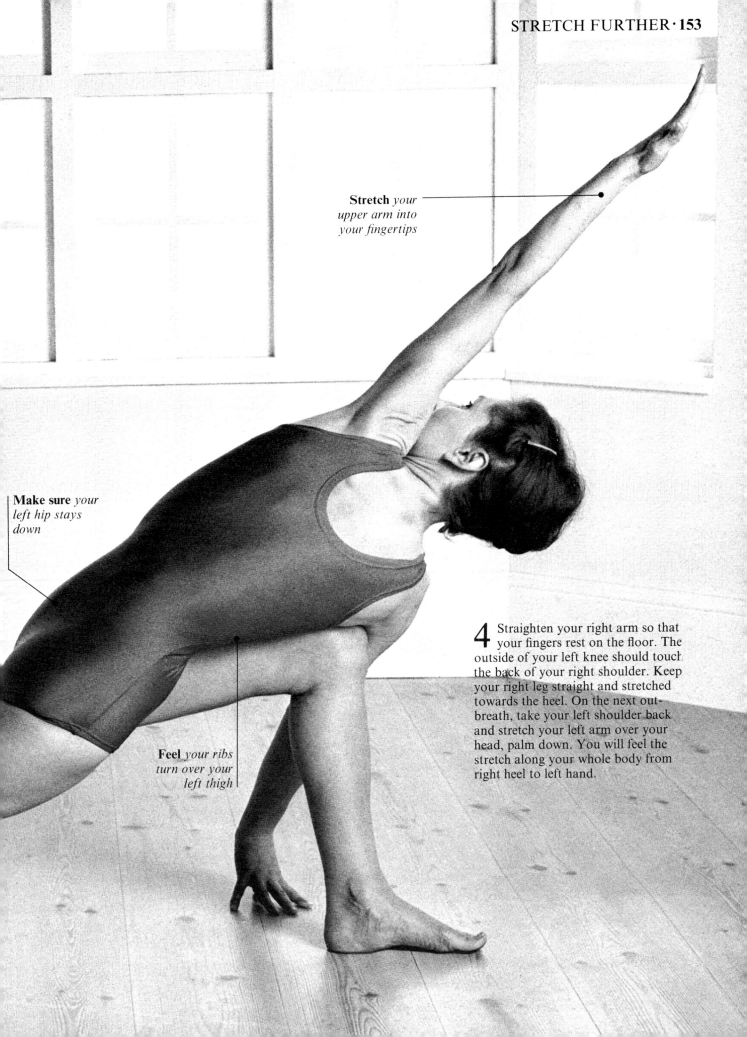

Stretch *your upper arm into your fingertips*

Make sure *your left hip stays down*

Feel *your ribs turn over your left thigh*

4 Straighten your right arm so that your fingers rest on the floor. The outside of your left knee should touch the back of your right shoulder. Keep your right leg straight and stretched towards the heel. On the next out-breath, take your left shoulder back and stretch your left arm over your head, palm down. You will feel the stretch along your whole body from right heel to left hand.

·BACKWARDS·

In these advanced stretches it is essential that the whole of the spine stretches as you extend backwards. You need to have flexible hips as well as shoulders and upper back, otherwise you will feel constricted at the waist.

First stretch

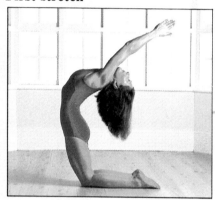 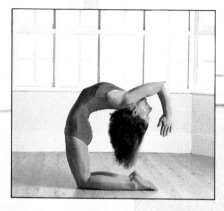

1 Kneel and stretch up as if preparing to do the basic stretch on p. 38. Taking your head back, lift up away from your hips, curving your upper back and opening your chest.

2 Let your arms bend as you continue to extend backwards. Keep your hips well forwards, with all your weight on your knees and feet. You should stretch slowly and with control.

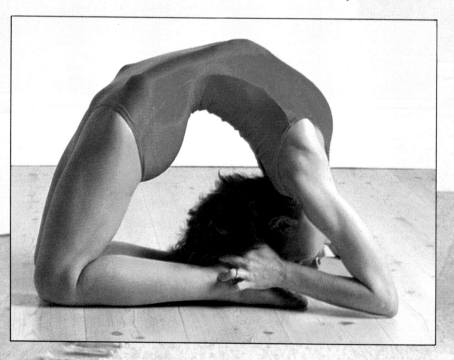

3 Catch your feet with your hands, your chest open and hips still forwards. Completely curve your spine so that your head rests on your feet with your elbows on the floor. Hold for a few seconds, then come up breathing in.

Second stretch

1 Lie on your front on a rug, right leg folded in front of you, left leg extended. Put your hands on the floor and lift up your trunk. Keep your hips straight so that your lower back is evenly stretched.

2 Bend your left leg. Breathing in, stretch your whole spine up and back. Stretch your right arm over your head and, on an out-breath, catch your left foot.

3 Keeping your left leg strong, take your left arm over your head and catch your foot. Breathing out, curve your upper back, extend your neck and take your head back until your foot is touching the top of your head. Hold for a few seconds, then let go of the foot one hand at a time. Breathe in and bring your head slowly up.

Stretch *your back foot*

Make sure *your right hip stays back*

Feel *your left hip come forwards*

Keep *the top of your knee flat on the floor*

·INDEX·

·ACKNOWLEDGMENTS·

Dorling Kindersley would like to thank the following for their special assistance: Jeff Veitch for the photography; Kris Watson for constructing the set; Adrian Ensor for the black and white prints; Karen Cochrane for the illustrations; Ken Hone for retouching; Chambers Wallace for typesetting; Richard and Hilary Bird for the index; Armstrong Flooring; Beverly of "Splitz"; Dr Cathy Bond; Alison Chappel; Christine Coleman; Dr Keith Fairweather; Fenwicks; Hilary Guy; Dr Faith Haddad; Nathalie of Joan Price's "The Face Place"; Pineapple; Dianne Scrivener.

· ABOUT · THE · AUTHORS ·

·MARY·STEWART·   ·MAXINE·TOBIAS·

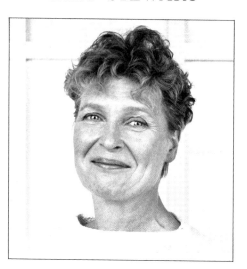 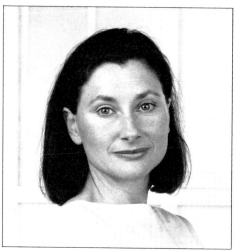

Maxine Tobias and **Mary Stewart** have been teaching yoga for more than fifteen years. Both took up yoga in the 1960s, practising on their own from books, and in 1969 they met in London on a teachers' training course. They studied the Iyengar method of yoga, under the supervision of B.K.S. Iyengar, one of the leading figures in yoga today. They then went on to study with Dona Holleman, a senior Iyengar teacher, in Italy and with Mr Iyengar himself in Poona, India.

In the 1970s they started training teachers together in London, serving on the committee for the B.K.S. Iyengar Teachers' Association. Together they held workshops and trained teachers at elementary and intermediate levels, their different teaching methods and approaches complementing each other.

Maxine Tobias has held relaxation workshops for physiotherapists and remedial gymnasts in a London teaching hospital. She holds classes for the Inner London Education Authority and also gives private tuition. She has contributed articles on yoga to a number of books and magazines.

Mary Stewart started off teaching in adult education institutes and now gives private lessons. She has taught in Italy and France. Among her special interests is teaching yoga for pregnancy and childbirth.

Both authors are refreshingly undoctrinaire in their approach. Dedicated though they are to yoga, they are firmly rooted in the traditions of Western culture and are committed to making a yoga-based exercise system accessible to everyone.

·AUTHORS'·ACKNOWLEDGMENTS·

We would like to thank Sri B.K.S. Iyengar of Poona, India for his generous teaching of yoga. His dedication to the subject has been a source of inspiration for us both. We would also like to thank Dona Holleman for sharing her knowledge with us and for encouraging us to work together. Our thanks also to Terry Tobias, Jane Beeson, Margaret Stokes, Madeleine Grove, Sarah Stirk and Eduardo for making so much effort to appear in the photographs, to Joan Price and Nathalie for the make-up and Beverly for making the leotards, Simon Stewart and Cathy Bond for reading the manuscript and making helpful criticisms. Many thanks to Jeff for taking the photographs even in times of adversity, Sybil for her patience and professional skill, Daphne for her expertise and Jane for her superb layouts, also Barbara without whose support none of this would have happened. Keith Stewart must be thanked for unfailing interest and patience over the two years it has taken to write *Stretch and Relax*.

Not to be forgotten, our pupils, who have always been so positive and encouraging about this book and, last but not least, the whole team at Dorling Kindersley for their unending courtesy, cheerfulness and enthusiasm, which have been of such help to us.